Musculoske Medicine in Clinical Practice

Musculoskeletal Medicine in Clinical Practice

John K. Paterson

With 24 Figures

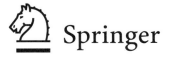 Springer

John K. Paterson, MBBS, MRCGP
Chairman, Scientific Advisory Committee, Federation Internationale de
Médecine Manuelle, 1990–1995; President, British Association of
Manipulative Medicine, 1986–1989; Hon. Sec. 1977–1985; Casualty
Officer, St Thomas' Hospital, 1951; Honorary Fellow, Federation
Internationale de Médicine Manuelle

British Library Cataloguing-in-Publication Data
A catalogue record for this book is available from the British Library

Library of Congress Control Number 2001012345

ISBN-10: 1-85233-966-7   Printed on acid-free paper
ISBN-13: 978-1-85233-966-1

Printed in the United States of America.   (BS/EB)

9 8 7 6 5 4 3 2 1   SPIN 11377283

Springer Science+Business Media
springeronline.com

◆

Dedicated to
all those who have sought to replace fantasy by fact
in this controversial field.

◆

Contents

Foreword ix

Preface xi

1 What Is Musculoskeletal Medicine? 1

2 The Scientific Bases of Musculoskeletal
   Medicine 9

3 The Patient's View of Musculoskeletal Medicine . . . 28

4 The Doctor's View of Musculoskeletal Medicine . . . 32

5 The Economics of Musculoskeletal Medicine 36

6 Teaching Musculoskeletal Medicine 40

7 Headache and Migraine 48

8 Neck Pain 55

9 Shoulder and Arm Pain 60

10 Chest Pain 63

11 Lower Trunk Pain 67

12 Pelvic Pain 72

13 Leg Pain 75

14 Will Musculoskeletal Medicine Work? 83

15 The Future of Musculoskeletal Medicine 86

Envoi 93

References 96

Further Reading 99

Glossary 101

Index 107

Foreword

Begin at the beginning and go on until you come to the end; then stop.
    Lewis Carroll (1832–1898), *Alice's Adventures in Wonderland*

This book does indeed begin at the beginning and lays a very firm foundation by not only clearly defining the subject, namely musculoskeletal medicine, but also stating what the text discusses.

Having prepared the ground in a business-like manner, the author approaches the subject in a precise and informative manner. This is all to the good, as there is a dearth of informed and informative works concerning this particular aspect of medical practice. Therefore, this book should be welcomed by all those for whom it is written, namely health care professionals and their patients.

Those who expect a textbook of practice will be disappointed. Whilst there is information aplenty, this is not a bench book; rather, it is a more leisurely guide to the clinical and administrative aspects of an important but neglected area of human suffering. The reader must appreciate that this book needs more than a single read-through. It should be read thoroughly and inwardly digested before either rushing to take up the cudgels of manipulation or to condemn the author roundly for propagating witch-doctoring.

However, the latter should not be undertaken lightly, for the author is a man of long experience in the field and is well known and respected for his sense and sensitivity. Before crossing swords with John Paterson, the tyro should be very sure of the facts upon which his adversarial conduct is placed. The end result will be such that one or more of the practices described herein would be extremely welcome.

Whatever the initial reaction, on more mature consideration it is soon realised that the trend running through this book is not only to inform but also to initiate thought and debate. It subserves this task well, and although not all readers will agree with all the diagnostic and therapeutic proposals, it will, undoubtedly, make people think, and with thought to see how they may change their practices to benefit their patients. Also, patients will gain some insight into the difficulties their doctors face and through this will be able to help themselves and their caregivers more effectively.

This is a well-referenced and readable book, with further reading indicated, together with a glossary. It is a well-constructed book, recommended to all who have interest in this aspect of medicine and to those who wish to learn more.

So to the end; but the end is really the beginning. More information will lead to better practice and more enquiry will lead to more practitioners adding further skills and expertise with which to benefit their patients. The patients, too, will imbibe knowledge of the problems associated with their treatment and be aware of the constraints applied to and impeding their helpers. What more can any reader ask for?

Dr. Keith Budd,
Menston, Ilkley, West Yorkshire

Preface

Musculoskeletal medicine is a term that has been introduced relatively recently. It has not as yet been really adequately defined, with the result that large numbers of both the medical profession and the public have become confused as to what it really is. This situation demands clarification. It is primarily involved with the study of pain perception and its modification, as well as the anatomy, physiology, and pathology of the skeleton and the muscular system, which inevitably includes the extremely complex neuromuscular control mechanisms. It necessarily involves the interaction between all these elements. It is secondarily the practice of a variety of simple therapies aimed at relieving pain and reducing disability. An understanding of the epidemiology of its various manifestations is imperative for all those working in this field.

This short book outlines 15 different aspects of musculoskeletal medicine. It is not intended to be a comprehensive text (and it is restricted almost exclusively to spinal concerns), but it does address some of the more important problems found in this controversial field, and it offers a number of more informative sources the interested reader may pursue at will.

Little is currently taught of the subject within orthodox medicine. In view of the very common incidence of musculoskeletal problems in the community, and the enormous potential savings likely to be derived from widespread adoption of musculoskeletal techniques, particularly in general practice, this reveals an unacceptable gap in medical training. Of fundamental concern to altering this situation is the manner in which the orthodox medical profession currently views musculoskeletal medicine. Four main attitudes are found.

Many doctors still regard musculoskeletal medicine as little more than a hoax, believing its component parts to be at best marginal, complementary, or alternative. They feel that it should be shunned by the orthodox establishment. In view of some of the outlandish claims made for it, this at first sight seems a perfectly reasonable view.

A considerable number, in some degree and perhaps reluctantly, recognise its uses (and its limitations), although they are not prepared to delve into it in depth, or to espouse it in public.

A small but growing number practice it to a varying extent, in a plethora of guises. In 2004 they remain a small percentage of the profession.

A proportion of the third group appears to have gone overboard in their somewhat uncritical acceptance of the tenets of the declared alternative ideologies, such as osteopathy and chiropractic, some of which have been shown not to have the benefit of scientific proof.

Observing the changing trends in the field over 40 years, I have come to the conclusion that the potential benefits to the patient that may be derived from a clearer understanding of the field throughout the medical profession are more than substantial – they are enormous. The most difficult question is how best to promote this. The chief obstacles to achieving such an understanding lie in the manner in which the field has been previously presented to the profession at large. To this end it is necessary to consider current attitudes, with a view to possibly changing them.

The first group mentioned very properly shows great caution in accepting an ideology (or rather a hodgepodge of somewhat similar, though sometimes conflicting ideologies) in the absence of valid supporting evidence. For them, the need is for presentation of such evidence as there is, in a sober, scientific manner. My aim here is to point them in the right direction for discovering such admittedly limited evidence as does exist.

The second group comprises those who are fundamentally perhaps less antipathetic toward musculoskeletal medicine, but who are similarly demanding of the production of valid evidence. They may be more ready to change their views and practices as a result of this demand being met. If such changes are to come about, they nonetheless need solid reassurance regarding the potential value and the remarkable safety of the therapeutic techniques of musculoskeletal medicine, in preference to their just being told they are wrong not to plunge into the not very clearly defined musculoskeletal melting pot.

The third group needs no persuasion, but they do need to standardise their teaching on a genuinely scientific basis, if they are to be generally accepted internationally.

The fourth group knows that it has the God-given truth. Those who "know" as a matter faith in so doing render themselves incapable of learning, and this will be crystal clear to doctors in groups 1 and 2 – the majority. As I see it, the confrontational approach adopted by some of this frankly prejudiced group virtually guarantees failure to change the minds of the bulk of the profession.

Some will view with suspicion the number of references to the work of Burn and myself. This is deliberate, not by way of self-advertisement, but rather because we offer over 1200 sources in the literature, supporting what we have written and taught over 17 or 18 years.

Is this short book of any value? Its chances of influencing group 4 are near to nil, but this does not matter in the slightest. It might prove of interest to group 3, and greater coordination internationally would certainly show the field in a better light. If it can reassure group 2, indeed it has real value. If it penetrates the perfectly understandable, deeply ingrained reservations of group 1, it will have made a substantial contribution to the well-being of a great many patients. But first it needs to be read – critically, but without too much bias! At the same time, a better informed public is likely to call for the changes necessary to achieve any real improvement in the current, very unsatisfactory situation.

I am deeply grateful to Dr. Keith Budd for his meticulous, positively critical comments on my original draft, and for his thoughtful foreword to this book.

Chapter 1
What Is Musculoskeletal Medicine?

Musculoskeletal medicine addresses pain perception and its modification, as well as the anatomy, physiology, and pathology of the skeleton and the muscular system, which inevitably includes the extremely complex neuromuscular control mechanisms. It involves the interaction between all these elements. Musculoskeletal medicine is secondarily the practice of a variety of simple therapies aimed at relieving pain, restoring normal posture and mobility, and reducing disability. An understanding of the epidemiology of its various manifestations is imperative for all those working in this field, and for the sufferers who currently are often ill-advised.

Little is currently taught of the subject within orthodox medicine. In view of the very common incidence of musculoskeletal problems and the enormous potential savings shown to be likely to be derived from the widespread adoption of musculoskeletal medicine, this gap in medical training is unacceptable. But many doctors still feel that it should be shunned by the orthodox establishment. In view of some of the outlandish claims made for it, this at first sight seems a perfectly reasonable view. Yet the potential benefits to the patient that may be derived from a clearer understanding of the field throughout the medical profession are enormous. But the patient, too, needs to distinguish between fact and fiction. The most difficult question is how best to promote such understanding. Too many people are saying conflicting things – with certitude! The arguments have been raging for many years, and still we do not have a consensus. First I present a number of proven facts and expose a few fantasies. The book should provoke the interest of the whole medical profession, though chiefly of general practitioners and medical educators, at the same time as encouraging the public to demand a better service.

EIGHTEEN FACTS REGARDING VERTEBRAL MANIPULATION

Unhappily, the 2001 conference on back pain at the Royal Society of Medicine (RSM) resulted in no decisions or resolutions. The following 18 facts remain of significance to a great many people. Each one is backed up by sound scientific evidence, for the reader's convenience to be found in a single reference volume (1):

1. Hippocrates used and taught vertebral manipulation, rendering it 100% orthodox within Western medicine.

2. This therapy was dropped by the medical profession for no clear reason, though possibly (in common with the introduction of the stethoscope) in an attempt to distance the physician from the patient, for fear of contagion.

3. Osteopathy originated in 1874 as a declared alternative to orthodox medicine, which latter its originator regarded as both wrong and dangerous. Its chief diagnostic base remains the identification of abnormal movement of individual vertebral joints, its chief therapy directed toward the restoration of normal movement.

4. It has been shown that the range of joint movement varies considerably from individual to individual and from one spinal level to another – *in the absence of pain.* Clinical identification of such "abnormalities," in addition to being a subjective impression, is clearly therefore of no diagnostic significance.

5. Chiropractic originated in 1895, again as a declared alternative to orthodox medicine, its clinical diagnostic base being primarily the identification of abnormal bony position, its therapeutic object being the restoration of normal alignment.

6. Symmetry of vertebral form is rare. Therefore, the examiner's subjective impressions of differences in "knobbiness" may reflect either bony asymmetry or bony misalignment, or both. From a scientific view, it is thus again of no diagnostic significance.

7. In spite of facts 1 and 2 cited above, the orthodox medical educators of the United Kingdom have long been reluctant to reinstate manipulative procedures into undergraduate or postgraduate teaching. Apart from an understandable desire not to further load their curricula, it seems likely that this has been in measurable degree due to the diagnostic claims and therapeutic aims referred to in facts 3 and 5, shown to be invalid in facts 4 and 6.

8. Over a number of years, osteopaths, chiropractors, the British Institute of Musculoskeletal Medicine (BIMM) and the Fédération Internationale de Médecine Manuelle (FIMM) have

made a generally confrontational attempt to get these invalid claims accepted by the orthodox medical profession, and for musculoskeletal medicine to be regarded as a medical specialty. In view of facts 4 and 6, it is difficult to entertain such proposals seriously.

9. Recently, both BIMM and FIMM have altered their statutes specifically so as to permit the admission of nonmedical members. This means that neither organisation is any longer exclusively representative of orthodox medicine.

10. There is, however, ample evidence that manipulative techniques commonly produce rapidly beneficial responses – *though nonetheless unpredictably* (in spite of some "alternative" teaching).

11. The dangers and contraindications related to these therapies are now well documented and are very simple to teach.

12. The claim that teaching needs to be lengthy and costly has been shown to be erroneous, when applied to orthodox doctors. With a suitable manual, stressing the contraindications, supplemented by brief practical courses, doctors may be taught to employ these therapies very quickly and at minimal cost – and with a high degree of safety.

13. Over 20% of the general practitioners' work load is related to spinal disorders. About 50% of medical students are destined for primary care. Few have any introductory teaching in this field.

14. The great majority of cases may be treated on presentation within primary care. While this initially entails an appreciable increase to the GP's work load, this is reversed rapidly by the commonly substantial reduction in follow-up appointments. The load is indeed lessened.

15. Advantages to the patient are four: the likelihood of more rapid relief from pain and disability, more rapid return to work, marked reduction in prescription charges or payments for alternative treatments, and reduction in waiting times for those few requiring referral. The latter is surely welcome news for hardpressed specialists.

16. The advantages to the employer are greater continuity of productivity, with less administrative frustrations in finding replacements for workers, or satisfying customers – reflected in increased profit margins.

17. The chief advantages to the taxpayer are two: reduction in sickness benefit payments and reduction in hospitalisation costs. These reductions are likely to be enormous.

18. The choice of the medical educator must surely lie in either abandoning the patient to practitioners frankly opposed to orthodox medical science or including the proven aspects of musculoskeletal medicine as an integral part of the orthodox curriculum.

An adequate understanding of musculoskeletal medicine must be based primarily on a sober, unbiased study of the subject, which concerns movement (including locomotion and gesture), arrested movement (which is posture), and the mode of treatment of many of their dysfunctions. Both are inevitably dependent on the proper functioning of the neuromuscular system, which lies at the heart of its clinical application. It does not include serious conditions better treated by orthopaedic surgery, for example, or any of the inflammatory diseases – the latter being the accepted province of rheumatology. In the event of the problem becoming chronic, the best therapeutic choice must be the multidisciplinary pain clinic.

What is the history of musculoskeletal medicine? The term has only come into widespread use relatively recently. Previously, malfunction of the musculoskeletal system was assessed and treated on a largely empirical basis, if treated at all, the chief, though not the sole, mode of treatment being manipulation, mostly of the spine. Diagnosis was widely variable and commonly fanciful, rather than being scientifically aligned – too often remaining the case today (1). This issue will be discussed in a later chapter. In spite of its having been used for many centuries, at some stage vertebral manipulation, the core therapy in this field, was dropped by the physicians and apothecaries of Western medicine, for no clear reason. It is tempting to suggest that, as in the case of the introduction of the stethoscope, this could have been in an attempt by the physician to avoid contagion from the patient. Whatever the reason, the result of the medical profession's turning its back on this type of therapy was to leave it in the hands of the bone setters. It is worth remembering that in many countries its practice remains largely informal, with no specific training or standards of competence being applied to those offering these therapies. Nonetheless, there is no reason to doubt that their results are not often excellent.

Between 1992 and 1997, as chairman of the Scientific Advisory Committee of the FIMM, I searched for consensus regarding the scientific bases and practices of musculoskeletal medicine amongst established teachers from 12 countries, making substantial progress before leaving the task in the hands of others

(2). So far as I am aware, such coordination has not yet been achieved (see Chapter 6). At the same time there has emerged in some countries a somewhat vociferous lobby in favour of recognition of musculoskeletal medicine as a medical specialty on its own merits. Apart from making international coordination in this field more difficult, this raises a fundamental question: What are the factors justifying the establishment of a new specialty? Of old, we had physicians, surgeons, and apothecaries – no finer definition of status within the medical profession.

In the past the demand for anaesthetists, pathologists, rheumatologists, orthopaedic surgeons, cardiovascular surgeons, and an ever-growing host of others arose from two complementary sources. First were the numerous scientific advances that have played so important a part in the evolution of 20th and 21st century Western medicine. Second was the inability of general physicians and surgeons to cope with such rapid and dramatic changes on the existing basis – a trend that today continues unabated. Further specialisation became necessary as each existing discipline required some of its members to know more and more about less and less, to employ ever more sophisticated technology, and at the same time to learn extremely complex new skills. The demand came from within the ranks of the specialist establishment, rather than the setting up of each new specialist field being in response to clamour from without. It is only of late that such isolation has been seen to be counterproductive.

But where do patients with musculoskeletal problems first present? In the great majority of cases, the answer is in what is now known as primary care. Indeed, the incidence of these very common problems is enormous, making up in excess of 20% of the GP's work load (3). The size of the problem is illustrated by the fact that, several years ago, Private Patients Plan (by no means the biggest insurer in the field) was spending in excess of £24 million per annum on spine-related problems (4).

Nonetheless, it is unfortunately true that the average general practitioner has had no undergraduate or postgraduate introduction to the field. Only in recent years has he had the freedom and some encouragement to refer these patients to people with non-medical training in manual therapies – to selected physiotherapists, osteopaths, chiropractors – or to local colleagues in the field. He may, of course, refer them to hospital outpatient departments. This is commonly a tediously slow process for the patient that should most often be quite unnecessary, and it is reflected in substantial increases in cost to the patient or taxpayer, while the length of hospital waiting lists inevitably increases.

Surely, if the criteria mentioned earlier are to be observed, two questions need to be addressed in relation to this field. First, are there currently valid scientific advances in musculoskeletal medicine to warrant its practice being directed into the necessarily "tunnel-vision" of specialism – with all that this implies? Second, are the requisite knowledge and associated skills complex or difficult to master? The answer to both these questions is a firm no (see Chapter 6).

What is required to resolve this situation? The answer is sixfold. First comes an understanding of the epidemiology of pain – today often misunderstood or unknown – particularly of back pain, at the very core of musculoskeletal medicine. Second must be a clear knowledge of the mechanisms of pain perception and its modification – in particular including referred pain and referred tenderness, and the psychology of pain. Third is a competent grasp of the relevant anatomy, some of which may surprise the newcomer to the field – in particular the realisation that our skeletons are virtually never symmetrically formed. Fourth is a basic knowledge of the relevant pathology. Fifth, and of the greatest importance of the six, comes an awareness of the contraindications to vertebral manipulation, coupled with their rigid observance. Sixth is the acquisition of a few basic diagnostic and therapeutic skills.

Stripped of the all-too-common "magic" image, eschewing cult, it is remarkable how easily competence in such practical skills can be gained. Indeed, it is my personal experience that, with the dedicated use of a suitable manual (5), and provided he or she can ride a bicycle and play a decent game of Ping-Pong, the average general practitioner can master the requisite skills in three $1^1/_2$-day courses. What is the relevance of the bicycle and Ping-Pong? They provide evidence of a level of neuromuscular coordination sufficient to enable the doctor to put into practice the modest skills he has learned – in safety. If he or she wishes to study the subject in greater depth, comprehensive coverage of the scientific bases of musculoskeletal medicine is readily available (6). If the general practitioner is able to learn the basic theory and practice of vertebral manipulation coupled with the associated local anaesthetic/steroid injections with such ease, it is clearly time to look objectively at several aspects of its application. Postgraduate courses devoting 280 hours to such study are clearly out of touch with reality (7).

From the point of view of the patient, while it is quite wrong for the doctor to predict outcome of such therapies (although there are those who do so with staunch conviction), the likelihood remains that their early deployment will result in early improvement (8). This likelihood has the advantage of affecting not only the duration and severity of the patient's symptoms, but his or her ability to earn a living. The latter is also good for the taxpayer on three fronts: in the removal of the need for an enormous number of expensive and possibly protracted investigations and therapies; in the reduction of pressure on hospital outpatient facilities and inpatient beds; and in a reduction in spending on sickness benefit, whilst also reducing the patient's payment of prescription charges (see Chapter 3).

Many are the descriptions of type of pain – aching, grinding, pricking, or stabbing, to mention but a few. And this is true regardless of the degree of pain felt by the individual. It may be useful here to remember that many patients use the word *acute* to mean severe, rather than of sudden onset, and use the word *chronic* to mean either severe or disabling, rather than ongoing. Such misuse may prove misleading. Further confusion may arise in patients' failure to appreciate the phenomenon of referred pain – they just know where it hurts. They must be told the truth about the reality that pain may arise far from where they feel it. It is common for patients to need elucidation on these points. Indeed this is an essential part of any acceptable musculoskeletal consultation – as much as it is of the medical consultation in general.

Coupled with pain, patients may suffer tenderness. Again it is vital for them to be alerted to the fact that tenderness, like pain, may be referred. It is surprising how many patients do not mention tenderness voluntarily; they often have to be asked as well as being provoked by the examiner's finger.

From the point of view of the doctor in primary care, two matters are of significance. First, the patient with a musculoskeletal problem can commonly be treated on presentation, or within a very short time, in the reasonable expectation of benefit in a high proportion of cases. While the doctor needs a few minutes' extra time at first contact with those patients, in fact clinical time is saved in the long run, as subsequent consultations will be less frequent, owing to the common efficacy of easily deployed manipulative manoeuvres or simple injections (8). Indeed, the initial increase in work load is in practice reversed – there is an overall diminution! Second, benefit is gained from a substantially reduced expenditure on referrals and, in dispensing practices, on drugs.

I will discuss these last two matters (and others) in greater detail in Chapters 3 and 4. But first to the scientific bases of musculoskeletal medicine: How much do we really know? How much current teaching is based on hypothesis masquerading as fact? These are the matters that should head the priority list of the General Medical Council, the Royal Colleges, and medical educators.

Chapter 2
The Scientific Bases of Musculoskeletal Medicine

Many doctors are taught by their mentors to believe that the proponents of musculoskeletal medicine are a bunch of crackpots, dedicated to a variety of philosophies that do not add up in a scientific environment. In particular, many of those charged with medical education view vertebral manipulation with serious misgivings, believing it to be commonly useless and sometimes dangerous. On the other hand, those already involved in this field only too often express their views in somewhat unscientific manner. It seems to me that both approaches need to be revised, if the patient is to receive the potential benefits of these quick, safe, simple, and commonly effective therapies. The only way of achieving this is to present to both antagonists and protagonists the admittedly limited amount of evidence that currently enjoys the benefit of scientific validation. Reception of this approach by both camps will be determined by the degree to which they already "know" they are right (9). It must be recognised that "negative" research, designed to show a belief to be wrong, is perfectly justifiable if "the investigator's bias and prejudice are put aside at the moment of interpretation" (10).

Before discussing this matter in detail, it is important for all to realise that in science there is no such thing as absolute truth. The "ideas" people propose hypotheses, they or others devise means of testing these hypotheses, as a result of which they are shown to be right or wrong – in the light of contemporary understanding. At any time later someone is quite likely to show that a particular conclusion was wrong – this is the only way scientific knowledge can advance. So people who declare they know the truth – and there are many who do within the medical profession, including members of the British Institute of Manipulative Medicine and the Fédération Internationale de Médecine Manuelle, in addition to those of nonmedical disciplines – have to provide sound evidence for their belief. More important, they must be prepared to change their stance when they are shown to be wrong. Scientific truth is, by its very nature, transient – dogged certitude is, without exception, contrary to science; it is essentially a matter of faith (9).

In view of the prevalence of musculoskeletal problems encountered in primary care, this educational void needs to be filled. An acceptable approach to musculoskeletal medicine must cover the subjects detailed in the previous chapter, the epidemiology of back pain, pain perception and its modification (including referred pain and tenderness and the psychology of pain), relevant anatomy, relevant pathology, and the indications and contraindications for vertebral manipulation. The last item demands a careful modification of standard history taking, as well as modification of data recording (11). Only when this is done is it permissible to proceed to the simple diagnostic and therapeutic techniques that will enable the clinician to take appropriate action – in safety and in reasonable expectation of such action proving useful. Unhappily, this logical sequence is not always followed.

It is perhaps encouraging that the Royal College of General Practitioners recognises the importance of the subject, at least some universities have the question under consideration, and the General Medical Council is well aware of the problems associated with frankly alternative approaches. In spite of this, few medical students learn much of the epidemiology of back pain, although it is summarised succinctly by Wood (3) and by Crombie (12), the latter particularly in respect to persistent pain.

Few grasp the importance of referred pain and tenderness. Its scale is enormous. Kellgren's (13) "football jersey" tells but a part of the story of dermatomal representation. It is a topographical guide to the relative concentration of the spinal nerve roots involved at any point on the body's surface. It is vital to remember that there is a wide overlap of nerve fibres of all types at each segmental level, both within the spinal cord and without, both up and down. Outside the spine, it has even been shown that nerves run relatively superficially from the thoracolumbar junction as far as the buttock (14), while pain arising in the cervical spine may mimic migraine, ear, nose, and throat problems, as well as ocular and dental problems (15). Anterior chest pain may arise in the spine (16), as may abdominal pain (15). This means that the sites of origin of pain and tenderness (and of paraesthesias), may be far removed from their sites of perception. It underpins the whole concept of referred pain and referred tenderness – vital to an understanding of musculoskeletal medicine – and is crucial to local examination.

It is perfectly acceptable to use such dermatomal depictions for the purpose of recording sites of pain and paraesthesia. Because of the normal overlap of supply, they do not accurately reflect the innervation of those areas.

Regardless of cause, pain perception in the first place requires a stimulus, followed by transmission along C fibres (as well as A-delta fibres) to the basal nucleus of the anterior horn of the spinal cord, where onward transmission to the brain is chemically promoted at its synapse – provided the initial stimulus is adequate and its transmission is not interfered with. In fact, the C fibres are accompanied in the same peripheral nerves by larger, A-beta fibres (ending at the same synapses), which, if simultaneously or subsequently stimulated, may inhibit the onward transmission of pain to the brain (6). Pain may also be mediated via the sympathetic nervous system. It follows that, if mechanoceptor end-organs in the immediate vicinity of pain end-organs are stimulated, pain perception is likely to be blocked at the anterior horn (17). This is the only mechanism of which we are currently sure whereby vertebral manipulation works. It was the late Professor Barry Wyke who so aptly branded manipulators "professional mechanoceptor stimulators." It is also important to remember that it is the speed of mechanoceptor stimulation that enhances the efficacy of vertebral manipulation, rather than its magnitude – due to accelerator effect (18). This fact is of great importance in practical teaching in the field (see Chapter 6).

The psychology of pain is also of relevance to musculoskeletal medicine. Again, acute pain behaves very differently from chronic pain. Its effective management is therefore different. Pain behaviours are established that demand a specific approach (19). The McGill Pain Questionnaire proves an invaluable aid in dealing with these problems (20). All too commonly is the term *psychosomatic pain* used in a somewhat derogatory way. If one takes the trouble to think about it, all pain is psychosomatic – it is the individual's psychological interpretation of some damage done to a part of his or her soma, unless transmission of the appropriate stimulus has been inhibited. The fact that aversive reactions to nociceptive stimuli may be demonstrated in unconscious patients reinforces the suggestion that pain would have been felt, if the psyche had not been deliberately suppressed (Fig. 2.1).

According to Bond (21), it is extremely important to appreciate the substantial psychological differences between acute and chronic pain, and the resultant need for different approaches. A clear understanding of this issue not only justifies but also

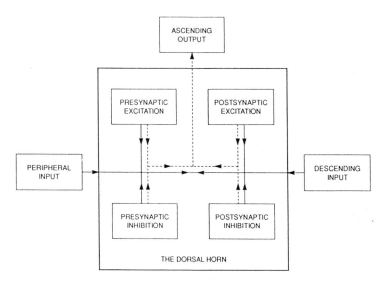

FIGURE 2.1. Acute pain mechanisms. (From Burn L, Paterson JK. *Musculoskeletal Medicine: The Spine*. London: Kluwer Academic Publishers, 1990, p. 46.)

demands the setting up of multidisciplinary pain clinics. So long as general practitioners do not commonly deal with these problems, such clinics are better equipped for their task if they have on their staff a clinician well versed in musculoskeletal medicine who may thereby counter the limitations of management of simple back pain in general practice (Fig. 2.2).

Every medical student learns anatomy. But there are some matters that need to be modified in current teaching, and a few need to be added. As far as the spine is concerned, the common idea that the intervertebral disc is primarily a weight-bearing structure needs to be abandoned. In fact, this is true for a remarkably small proportion of one's life. And if one considers mammalian species in general (of generally similar basic construction), one seldom finds protracted discal weight-bearing at all. Indeed the earliest mammals had spines that for long periods of time were at about 45 degrees from the vertical, and while the horse and the cow dropped the front end to become more or less spinally horizontal, humans went in the opposite direction and stood up – when they were not sitting or lying down! They remain in a minority!

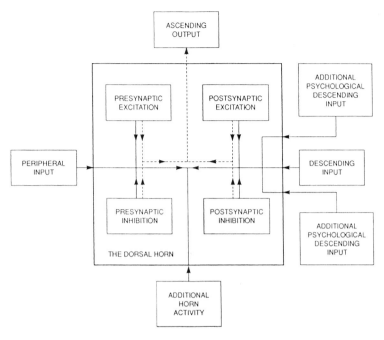

FIGURE 2.2. Chronic pain mechanisms. (From Burn L, Paterson JK. *Musculoskeletal Medicine: The Spine*. London: Kluwer Academic Publishers, 1990, p. 46.)

In fact, to use an engineering analogy, the intervertebral disc is part of a universal joint, of very little range, holding its parts together, as much as separating them, having a primarily cushioning effect. As the nucleus pulposus (like any other liquid or semiliquid) is incompressible, such cushioning can only be effected by stretching the annulus fibrosus and its supporting ligaments, simultaneously distorting the nucleus pulposus in all three dimensions. Likewise, movement is possible only on such asymmetrical stretching. Of course, in spite of common references to its supposed occurrence, dating only from 1932 in a report on a single case (22), and carried on for many years (23), the disc does not slip. Neither does disc protrusion simply arise from too great intradiscal pressure due to maintaining the upright posture; one of the commonest species to suffer from it is the dachshund (Fig. 2.3).

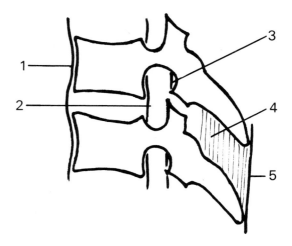

1. Anterior longitudinal ligament
2. Posterior longitudinal ligament
3. Ligamentum flavum
4. Interspinous ligament
5. Supraspinous ligament

FIGURE 2.3. The mobile segment. (From Paterson JK, Burn L. *An Introduction to Medical Manipulation*. Lancaster, England: MTP Press, 1985, p. 133.)

Clearly, the primary fault in disc protrusion must lie in the closely applied joint capsules and supporting ligaments, each known to have a rich nerve supply (24). So the continuing argument as to whether or not the annulus fibrosus has a nerve supply of its own is of little clinical consequence. If one is overstretched, the others are overstretched, too. It is also important to remember that no vertebra is ever perfectly symmetrical in form – a fact underlying the absolute necessity for all those of scientific bent to reject the diagnostic basis of chiropractic.

A further anatomical point of importance is that no spinal joint ever moves in isolation. Even at a single mobile segment (which also never moves on its own), in the absence of bony fracture, movement between two adjacent vertebrae is necessarily accompanied by movement at both the intervertebral and the posterior vertebral (or facet) joints. And the characteristics of all three movements are dissimilar – in different planes, in different directions, and to different degrees. The commonly taught concepts of detecting or provoking movement in a single spinal joint (25) are no more than fantasy. I do not intend to discuss peripheral joints in this book, but it is clear that the differing patterns to be found in the cervical, thoracic, lumbar, and pelvic joints must determine both their physiological and pathological movement.

Of particular importance to the manipulator is the detailed anatomy of the odontoid process of the second cervical vertebra. Laxity of the various ligaments holding this bony prominence in place puts the spinal cord at risk of compression, and it is the more important in view of the fact that rheumatoid arthritis not uncommonly weakens the odontoid process, but may also weaken its restraining ligaments, putting the patient at risk from cervical manipulation, which is absolutely contraindicated in this circumstance (Fig. 2.4).

Another small detail of anatomy is of the gravest importance: the course of the vertebral arteries in association with the first and second cervical vertebrae. This is tortuous, with the arteries passing through the transverse processes of the first cervical vertebra. The result of this is that extreme positioning, particularly in rotation of the cervical spine in extension, may cause occlusion of one artery by kinking. While of no particular importance in itself, as they are in effect joined within the skull, if the other vertebral artery happens to be blocked (perhaps by atheroma), then serious damage may result from such positioning, if prolonged. Unfortunately, relatively few manipulators are aware of this potential danger. This, together with the odontoid process and its supporting ligaments, will be considered in Chapters 7 to 13 (Fig. 2.5).

A further difficulty presents itself in the assessment of musculoskeletal problems: the phenomenon of muscle substitution. As has been shown by Basmajian and DeLuca (26), damage to the nerve supply of a number of muscle bundles automatically results in activation of other muscle bundles that until then were not activated, not necessarily in the same muscle. In practice, and in spite of common claims to the contrary, this often makes it clinically impossible to identify with certainty the specific muscle at fault.

I deliberately do not discuss biomechanics in this short, introductory book, because, while it is an interesting academic subject, according to Panjabi (27) it is of little significance to the primary care physician. However, there are many who take the opposite view, emphatically supported by Bogduk (28), that biomechanics is of great importance to the clinician. What seems

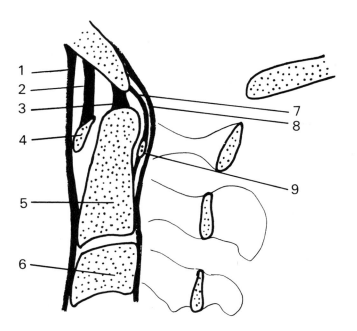

1. Anterior longitudinal ligament
2. Anterior occipitoatlantal membrane
3. Apical ligament
4. Anterior arch of atlas
5. Odontoid process
6. Vertebral body – C3
7. Occipitotransverse ligament
8. Median occipitoatlantal ligament – posterior longitudinal
9. Transverse ligament

FIGURE 2.4. The odontoid process. (From Paterson JK, Burn L. *An Introduction to Medical Manipulation*. Lancaster, England: MTP Press, 1985, p. 134.)

certain is that accurate measurement of the various factors is of little significance, if it is not known how to identify the normal. I leave it to the reader to make up his or her mind.

The question of x-rays in musculoskeletal medicine is vexing. Some practitioners (in particular chiropractors) demand routine pretreatment x-rays, which may demonstrate differences in bony contour and thereby assumed differences in bony position (29). In view of the fact that individual vertebrae are virtually never

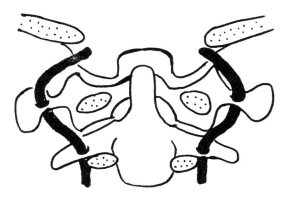

FIGURE 2.5. The course of the vertebral arteries. (From Paterson JK, Burn L. *An Introduction to Medical Manipulation*. Lancaster, England: MTP Press, 1985, p. 135.)

perfectly symmetrical (30), this observation can be misleading. Indeed, for this reason alone, to interpret such findings as evidence of bony malposition is unsound, and therefore it is not a valid indicator for specific manipulative therapy. Taking another x-ray immediately following manipulation may show changes in juxtaposition of adjacent vertebrae, but assessment of efficacy must still depend primarily on local, clinical examination and patient report.

"Functional" x-rays (25), in which serial images are taken in varying spinal positions (with the patient standing, sitting, or lying down), permit varying interpretations. It is, of course, true that x-rays may reveal the presence of scoliosis, osteophytes, rheumatoid arthritis, Schmorl's nodes, bony fracture, or secondary carcinoma, but most of these conditions may escape detection in their early stages, and it is highly significant that the Clinical Standards Advisory Group (CSAG) report on back pain recommends plain x-ray in simple back pain "if there are suspicious clinical features, or if pain has not settled in six weeks" (31). It is true that magnetic resonance imaging or other sophisticated investigation is likely to reveal more, but this is for consideration by the specialist rather than by the general practitioner. There is nothing unorthodox in any of these matters!

There is yet another problem in the justification of vertebral manipulation as an orthodox therapy. On the whole, justification of any therapy is best founded on prior diagnosis, coupled with safety. But specific diagnosis is seldom possible in this field.

Nonetheless, vertebral manipulation is acceptable in cases of simple back pain, or in cases of referred pain, *in the absence of contraindications*, so long as it is abandoned early in the face of poor response, in favour of a different therapy or hospital referral. If the majority of cases of simple back pain continue to be referred to hospital, the waiting lists can only remain unacceptable. And, of course, a large increase in the use of x-rays (particularly lumbar ones, which account for about two thirds of the total incidence), inevitably carries an additional radiation risk to the patient.

One of the problems in this field is the number of diagnoses to be found in identical circumstances – they cannot all be right! Bone out of place, solitary blocked joint, and sacroiliac maladjustment are offered as examples, each said to justify specific procedures. This highlights the importance of local examination as an addition to orthodox orthopaedic and neurological examination, and the employment of gentle, nonspecific procedures that do not hurt the patient. Contrary to widespread teaching, there is no such thing as a specific vertebral manipulation. Unhappily, there is at present a paucity of satisfactory clinical trials of both efficacy and safety. One reason for this is the difficulty in making a definitive clinical diagnosis in the majority of cases, for example, beyond the "simple back pain" of the CSAG report (31), so that comparisons may not be between like and like (see Chapter 6). What seems inescapable is that empiricism must play a part in this field, and that this is perfectly acceptable, provided that the doctor is honest in admitting this and rigidly observes the contraindications described.

Although posture has never been adequately identified as an epidemiological cause of spinal pain (except in extreme cases), it is important to note it, in case of posttherapeutic change. Basic movements should also be included, noting both differences in range of flexion, extension, side bending, and rotation, and at the same time noting which movements provoke exacerbation of the patient's pain. Graphical recording of results saves time and affords rapid recall at subsequent examinations. An acceptably comprehensive yet simple example of this is to be found later in this chapter. Such recall may be similarly achieved with suitable software design in the event of records being computerized. It is vital to regard local examination, at all segmental levels, as an addition to orthopaedic or neurological examination but never as a substitute.

In both history taking and in local examination an enormous amount of time may be saved by such standardised data recording. There are four advantages to this. First, a suitably designed form reduces the likelihood of the doctor forgetting a detail that might prove vital. Second, the majority of entries are by a checkmark, cross, or slash, rather than by more time-consuming longhand entries. Keying information directly into a computer is likely to further reduce the time needed, once a suitable programme has been evolved. Third, whether manually or on screen, at each review of the patient, all necessary information is readily at hand. Fourth, recording of the work of different doctors becomes immediately comparable for research purposes. It is important that such a data recording form avoid the use of theoretical diagnoses (such as a solitary joint being mechanically blocked) and imaginary therapeutic procedures (such as putting a bone back into place). Since 1983, with the helpful criticism of many postgraduate students, Burn and I have evolved a system that works well with minimal additional demands on time, as there is relatively little need for words to be written, and a checkmark, cross, or slash is much quicker to make. Originally formally presented to the profession in 1986 at an international congress in Madrid, it has seen numerous improvements (11).

On the first page, apart from identification data, there is a reminder of the 12 most important contraindications to manipulation. Site and radiation of pain are recorded by reference to the chart of dermatomal innervation already given, as is site of paraesthesias and numbness, either left or right. Intensity of pain is entered as slight, moderate, or severe, by +, ++, or +++. Otherwise entry of data is self-explanatory. It allows for recording of data on three occasions. On the reverse side of the form, differences in global movements are recorded with a dash across each of the diagrammatic lines – one for slight, two for moderate, and three for severe. Pain provoked by these movements is similarly recorded by crosses – one for slight, two for moderate, and three for severe. Positive traditional signs are recorded by a plus in the appropriate box. Positive local signs are recorded as are the site of pain – by reference to the dermatomal innervation. A positive sign relating to the anterior branch of the 5th cervical nerve on the right will be entered simply as C5A in the right-hand box, a posterior referral on the left as C5P (Figs. 2.6 and 2.7).

Posture and global movements are included chiefly as a means of judging progress, rather than as diagnostic aids. To complement the history, the doctor needs to learn no more than seven (additional) diagnostic techniques: skin pinching, search for muscle guarding and trigger points, eliciting pain on serial segmental sagittal pressure or vertebral rotation, search for

MUSCULOSKELETAL CASE ANALYSIS SHEET

Patient's name...Serial No:........................

Address ....

....Phone ....

Date of birth   /   /   Male:............. Female.......... Insurance.......................

Contraindications: Fractures....... Neoplasm........ Scheuermann........ A/spondylitis......
Polymyalgia........ Osteoporosis........ Rh.A. of neck........ Basilar insuff........ Grisel......
Myelopathy........ Sphincter problems........ Saddle anaesthesia........

HISTORY – Present episode

Subject report		/ /		/ /		/ /	
		L	R	L	R	L	R
Pain –	Site						
	Radiation						
	Intensity						
	Duration						
	Worsened by						
	Improved by						

Altered sensation

	P & N						
	Numbness						

Activities of daily living

	Hoovering						
	Bedmaking						
	Ablutions						
	Cooking						
	Ironing						
	Putting on socks						
	Shopping						
	Gardening						
	Sports						
	Sitting at desk						
	Other work						
	Road/rail travel						
	Air travel						

Pain behaviour

	Pill taking habit						
	Other treatments						
	Hours in bed per 24						
	Forced absenteeism						
	Litigation pending						

Previous episodes

Year .... Site ....Duration in days............. weeks ....months ....
Therapy ....Outcome ....
Year .... Site ....Duration in days............. weeks ....months ....
Therapy ....Outcome ....
Relevant medical history ....
....
Affect ....

FIGURE 2.6. Data recording sheet – obverse. (From Paterson JK. *Vertebral Manipulation: A Part of Orthodox Medicine*. London: Kluwer Academic Publishers 1995, p. 32.)

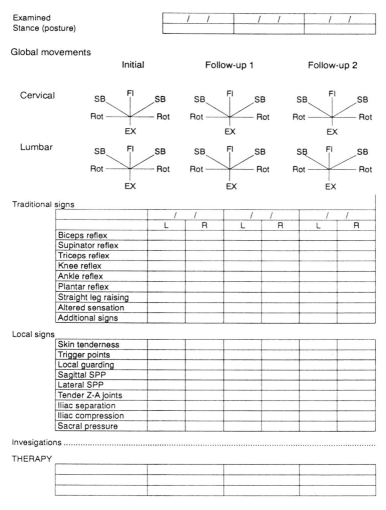

Examined	/	/	/	/	/	/
Stance (posture)						

Global movements

| | Initial | Follow-up 1 | Follow-up 2 |

Cervical

Lumbar

Traditional signs

	/	/	/	/	/	/
	L	R	L	R	L	R
Biceps reflex						
Supinator reflex						
Triceps reflex						
Knee reflex						
Ankle reflex						
Plantar reflex						
Straight leg raising						
Altered sensation						
Additional signs						

Local signs

Skin tenderness					
Trigger points					
Local guarding					
Sagittal SPP					
Lateral SPP					
Tender Z-A joints					
Iliac separation					
Iliac compression					
Sacral pressure					

Invesigations ....

THERAPY

FIGURE 2.7. Data recording sheet – reverse. (From Paterson JK. *Vertebral Manipulation: A Part of Orthodox Medicine*. London: Kluwer Academic Publishers 1995, p. 33.)

zygoapophyseal tenderness, and three pelvic tests. Most of these are illustrated below (Figs. 2.8 to 2.14).

By combining the information derived from these tests, physicians will be in a position to decide where to apply their chosen therapeutic choice (see Chapter 6). To make this clearer,

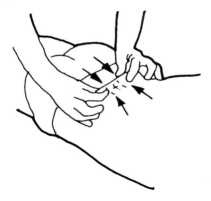

FIGURE 2.8. Skin tenderness. (From Paterson JK. *Vertebral Manipulation: A Part of Orthodox Medicine*. London: Kluwer Academic Publishers 1995, p. 39.)

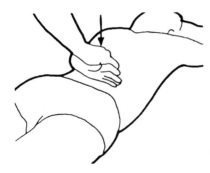

FIGURE 2.9. Sagittal spinous process pressure (SPP). (From Paterson JK. *Vertebral Manipulation: A Part of Orthodox Medicine*. London: Kluwer Academic Publishers 1995, p. 41.)

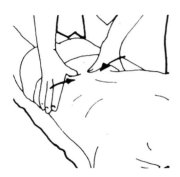

FIGURE 2.10. Lateral spinous process pressure. (From Paterson JK. *Vertebral Manipulation: A Part of Orthodox Medicine*. London: Kluwer Academic Publishers 1995, p. 42.)

FIGURE 2.11. Tenderness of zygoapophyseal joints. (From Paterson JK. *Vertebral Manipulation: A Part of Orthodox Medicine*. London: Kluwer Academic Publishers 1995, p. 43.)

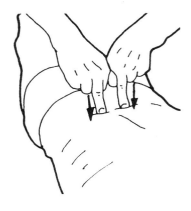

FIGURE 2.12. Iliac separation. (From Paterson JK. *Vertebral Manipulation: A Part of Orthodox Medicine*. London: Kluwer Academic Publishers 1995, p. 44.)

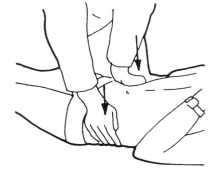

FIGURE 2.13. Iliac compression. (From Paterson JK. *Vertebral Manipulation: A Part of Orthodox Medicine*. London: Kluwer Academic Publishers 1995, p. 44.)

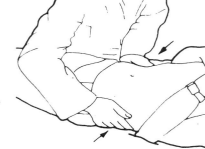

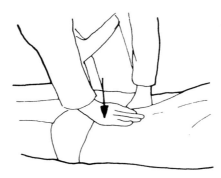

FIGURE 2.14. Sacral thrust. (From Paterson JK. *Vertebral Manipulation: A Part of Orthodox Medicine*. London: Kluwer Academic Publishers 1995, p. 45.)

an example is given of a completed data recording sheet (Figs. 2.15 and 2.16).

The example of a completed data recording sheet is offered to illustrate how simple it is to make detailed recordings and to retrieve information from it. Similar considerations apply in the event of the record being transferred to disc. Aside from the personal identification entries, at the first consultation this patient's history is seen to reveal severe left-sided head and shoulder pain over the preceding 3 weeks, worsened by movement but improved by analgesics, with no pins-and-needles sensation or numbness. There are no remarks as to contraindications. As for activities of daily living, vacuuming was a major problem; bed making, washing, and shopping were moderate problems; and cooking, ironing, and sitting at a desk were minor problems. The patient's sole treatment was Distalgesic × 2 four times a day. She spent 7 hours a day in bed, and had lost 2 days from work. Litigation was not being considered. In 1969 she had low back pain for 3 months, for which she had had bed rest and analgesics. This was following a heavy fall from a horse. She had had no scanning investigations. She had had no recurrence until this episode.

Initial examination is seen to show normal posture, with minor restriction of cervical movement in extension, moderate restriction in rotation to the left and in side bending to the right. In response to traditional examination, she showed no abnormality.

MUSCULOSKELETAL CASE ANALYSIS SHEET

Patient's name... *Mrs Rosemary BLOGGS* ....Serial No: *F 523/*
Address... *3, Treelined Avenue* ....Insurance.. *BUPA*
.... *West Homersham, Hants* ....Phone. *5290 17692/*
Date of birth *14 / 01 / 42*   Male.... Female. *✓*

Family doctor's name... *H. Fernandez* ....
Address... *The Health Centre, High Street* ....
.... *West Homersham* ....Phone. *5290 671426* ..NHS/Private. *N* ...

HISTORY - Present episode.

Subject report		23 /01/ 89		30 /01/ 89		/ /	
		L	R	L	R	L	R
Pain –	Site	Head A					
	Radiation	Shoulder					
	Intensity	Severe					
	Duration	3/52					
	Worsened by	Moving					
	Improved by	Analg.					
Altered sensation							
	P & N	o					
	Numbness	o					

Activities of daily living

	Hoovering	Major					
	Bedmaking	Moderate					
	Ablutions	Moderate					
	Cooking	Minor					
	Ironing	.					
	Putting on socks	O					
	Shopping	Moderate					
	Gardening						
	Sports·						
	Sitting at desk	Minor					
	Other work						
	Road/rail travel						
	Air travel						

Pain behaviour

	Pill taking habit	Distalgesic × 2 yds		o	
	Other treatments			o	
	Hours in bed per 24	7		7	
	Forced absenteeism	2/7			
	Litigation pending	No			

Previous episodes
    Year. *1969* . Site. *LBP* ...... Duration Days... Weeks. *3* . Months....
    Therapy *Bed + Analgesics* .... Outcome *No recurrence since* ..
    Year...... Site......... Duration Days... Weeks... Months....
    Therapy...........................Outcome..................

Relevant medical history... *1969 - Heavy fall from horse* ....

Investigations... *o* ....

FIGURE 2.15. Example of data recording – obverse. (From Burn L, Paterson JK. *Musculoskeletal Medicine: The Spine*. London: Kluwer Academic Publishers, 1990, p. 164.)

In response to local examination, she showed skin tenderness anteriorly on the left side at the C4 level, local guarding of the paravertebral muscles on the left at the same level, and tenderness over the left C4-5 zygoapophyseal joint.

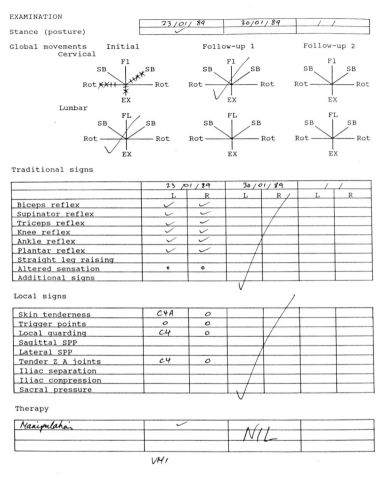

FIGURE 2.16. Example of data recording – reverse. (From Burn L, Paterson JK. *Musculoskeletal Medicine: The Spine*. London: Kluwer Academic Publishers, 1990, p. 165.)

This appreciable amount of information derived from examination of posture, movement, and the local physical signs is recorded by no more than five lines, five crosses, two checkmarks, five zeroes, and three small groups of letters and figures. Therapy is recorded by a single word and a checkmark, its immediate result by one group of three letters. Follow-up 1 week later is recorded by 3 checkmarks and the word *nil*.

It will at once be seen that such a method has the twin advantages of rapidity of both entry and recall, which contributes to a saving of time for the practitioner (over and above the substantial time saved by the likely reduction in the number of follow-up visits required).[1] Apart from the added notes item, it affords the further advantage of similarity of mode of recording, which is of value from a research point of view in comparison of results from different practitioners.

[1]In the UK, visit implies a domiciliary visit, whereas attendance is more commonly referring is seeing a patient in the surgery/office.

Chapter 3
The Patient's View of Musculoskeletal Medicine

As in any other area of clinical medicine, the patient is the most important person in the world. And so he or she should be! Far more so than administrative goals, targets, or other inanimate objects. After defining musculoskeletal medicine and offering a scientifically acceptable basis for its reinstatement within conventional medicine, we now consider the patients. What do they want? What do they need? What may they expect from a comprehensive health service? They usually want to be free of pain and any accompanying disability. Their particular need is to resume their normal way of life, the requirements for achieving this being widely variable. What they may expect from the National Health Service (NHS) will be discussed later.

So first let us look at the patients' current, unsatisfactory state. Foremost, they complain of pain. Limitation of spinal movement often accompanies pain, either because there appears to be a mechanical block, or because movement, in one direction or another, exacerbates the pain, or as a result of muscle spasm itself often causing pain. This may present as a disturbance of posture, of gait, or of other attempted movement. Inevitably it constitutes a disability. The patients are prevented from performing to their accustomed standard – at work, at play, or in bed. Of fundamental importance is the fact that such limitation is related to the individual patient's normal performance – and no one has yet discovered a means by which this can be satisfactorily measured clinically. Of course, apart from the inconvenience of not being able to enjoy their other pursuits, this often results in loss of earnings. The sickness certificate may at first sight seem a blessing, but the earliest possible relief from symptoms is of far greater value. Patients want to see the end of their symptoms quickly and to resume their normal lifestyle.

And here arises a matter of the greatest importance. Many patients have been brought up to believe that they should be told what is wrong with them before being treated. Many doctors and other health care workers share the same superficially attractive view. At the present time, within the broad practice of musculoskeletal medicine, numerous different diagnoses are applied to identical patterns of symptoms and physical signs. While perhaps expecting a diagnosis, the patient has no way of anticipating the likelihood of one diagnosis or another being right! There are too many on offer, and a wise choice is difficult. This feature is outlined in the brief statement of 18 facts to be found in Chapter 1. For example, osteopaths often refer to restriction of movement of a particular joint being at the root of the trouble, for which they suggest restoration of the "normal" range by mobilisation or manipulation (25). Chiropractors commonly put the problem down to a bone being out of place, declaring their intention of "putting it back" (29). A large proportion of doctors still believe in protrusion of an intervertebral disc as being a common cause of these problems, a surprising number still clinging to the outmoded concept of a disc having slipped (23). And there is a substantial collection of further diagnoses to be found, few with the advantage of scientific validation. This is, indeed, a recipe for confusion, if not for disaster.

In spite of this very unsatisfactory situation, in my personal experience there are few patients who will not accept a rational explanation as to what appears to be the site of origin of their pain, coupled with the honest admission that it is seldom possible to make a definitive diagnosis (see Chapter 2).

The result of the current welter of diagnoses is to confuse the patients – whom are they to believe? So the treatment they receive depends on two factors – which of the many diagnoses sounds most reasonable to them and whom they consult – or perhaps in the reverse order. This opens up the ongoing debate over conventional and complementary medicine. For a good many years, consulting a conventional doctor has been synonymous with bed rest and analgesics (taken orally or injected), perhaps some form of physiotherapy, a sickness certificate, and waiting for nature to take its course – in letting the pain just go away. In the more extreme cases it has meant undergoing a variety of tests, followed by surgical intervention of one sort or another, with surprisingly variable and not wholly predictable results. Oddly enough, in spite of Hippocrates having used and taught it, vertebral manipulation has been for many years very seldom considered within conventional Western medicine. This situation is slowly changing, but general medical acceptance of musculoskeletal medicine is painfully slow – literally!

For a long time after conventional medicine abandoned vertebral manipulation (for no known reason), patients had little alternative but to accept their doctor's limited management, put up with their pain, or consult a bone setter. These totally untrained, unqualified practitioners seem to have satisfied a great many patients – indeed it was their frequent success in cases in which I had failed that first provoked me into taking an interest in the field. In rural areas numerous patients still go to the local bone setter, in preference to the doctor. Then came osteopathy – presented by Andrew Taylor Still, an American Army doctor, in frustration and despondency over his family's experiences with orthodox medicine, who "turned to God and religion" (32) as an alternative. Not many years later chiropractic was introduced by Daniel David Palmer, a teacher turned grocer, believed to have the gift of healing (29). The patient's choice was in this way substantially extended, now with what sounded more like logical diagnoses. Once again, the treatments commonly proved very useful in musculoskeletal problems, and showed remarkable practical similarities, in spite of the practitioners' widely differing ideologies. And, over the past century and more, these prototype complementary disciplines became more refined, spawning further and more specific diagnoses. But the underlying confusion remained and deepened.

Perhaps the most unsatisfactory aspect of this situation was that practitioners of all persuasions often made predictions as to what was likely to happen to the patient. Many still do, and at the same time many patients expect a definitive prognosis. It is now clear that few musculoskeletal therapies are susceptible to prediction of outcome (31). Some practitioners decry this (together with the common lack of a definitive diagnosis) as amounting to a contraindication to their use. To my mind, any prediction is subject to doubt, and there is nothing wrong with empiricism, so long as the doctor is honest enough to admit to its use and cautious enough to respect the very real contraindications to the use of particular treatments. So the patient assured of a diagnosis and offered a prediction of outcome of therapy should be especially on his guard (see Chapter 14).

If patients (in the United Kingdom) opt for treatment under the National Health Service, they are likely to face an unacceptable delay in being treated. As in the case of many other subspecialty areas, patients are unlikely to be seen initially by a doctor with training in musculoskeletal medicine. Even if seen soon, unless exempt, they will have to pay a substantial prescription charge, as well as facing loss of earnings. In my experience (although I certainly do not recommend it), if patients go to the bone setter, they will pay a much smaller fee than they would have done for their drugs (after a negligible wait), with reasonable expectation of substantial and rapid improvement. If patients consult an osteopath or chiropractor, they will pay a higher fee, but the clinical prospects may be rather better. If the doctor is one of the few with training in musculoskeletal medicine, patients have a good chance of having the pain resolved and returning to work – often at no cost whatever (8). If they choose to seek help from one of the slowly growing number of doctors practising privately in this field, they are likely to find very much higher fees to be met, often unacceptable in the absence of health insurance cover, sometimes unacceptable to the Provident Associations also.

Of course, it is up to the patients to make the important decision as to whom to consult, dependent on the factors noted in the preceding paragraph and the availability of a suitable service readily at hand. But patients must accept that, whatever claims may be made to the contrary, no one can tell whether or not any one treatment will work for them (31). There is little wrong with empiricism, so long as the physicians know this to be, at times and to a varying extent, the basis of their choice of treatment, and so long as they explain this to the patient and rigidly respect the contraindications to vertebral manipulation. It would seem that the prospect for the patient is rosy, indeed, once the orthodox medical profession takes on this challenge.

Chapter 4
The Doctor's View of Musculoskeletal Medicine

In this field, most doctors in the United Kingdom fall into one of two camps. The majority still regards musculoskeletal medicine as complementary at best, only relatively few recognising its full potential value. Of more serious import, a substantial number believe its limited therapies to be useless, a proportion of them viewing its chief therapy, vertebral manipulation, as intrinsically dangerous. I hope to persuade them that, in the light of the evidence currently available, these views are outdated. As mentioned earlier, Hippocrates used and taught vertebral manipulation, making it difficult for today's teachers to justify its being presented as an alternative – surely with its ancient history it has to be 100% orthodox. Of course, its ancient history has little bearing on its value, but we need good reason to justify having dropped it. To date I have found none.

Whether they are aware of the fact or not, the doctors who see the greatest number of musculoskeletal problems are the general practitioners; with the exception of those patients who elect to go directly to truly complementary practitioners, primary care usually remains the first port of call for them (3). Bone setters still ply their trade in rural areas, and there are considerable numbers of practitioners who describe themselves as osteopaths or chiropractors, some of them without benefit of proper qualifications. But how many general practitioners today have the training adequate to practice musculoskeletal procedures in safety? And how many can find the necessary time to enable them to pursue such a course?

Clinical recognition of these all-too-common problems must come primarily from a thorough understanding of the relevant history, in particular in respect to the differences between acute and chronic pain. Doctors must learn to ask the right questions, in order to determine whether they are dealing with simple back pain or something more sinister. It is important to have detailed information about previous attacks, their severity, their course, their treatment, and its result. It is vital to determine any contraindications to vertebral manipulation, or indications for other forms of treatment, most of these being discovered on taking an adequate history, rather than on local examination. It is here that the "red flags" of the Clinical Standards Advisory Group (CSAG) report are of the greatest value (31). These red flags include sphincter problems.

It must be remembered that, just as in the universally accepted referral of pain of spinal origin to the leg – everyone knows about sciatica arising in the spine – similar referral takes place both anteriorly and posteriorly to the pelvis, the abdomen, the thorax, the shoulders, the arms, the neck and the face and head (the latter including such symptoms as tinnitus and vertigo). Details of these matters will be found in later chapters. It must be stressed that taking a full history does not take very long, provided the doctor works to a consistent pattern, preferably using a standardised data recording form. One such form is illustrated in Chapter 2.

Local examination, in addition to asking the appropriate questions of the patient, often reveals asymmetrical local physical signs. Patients do not always volunteer information about differences in sensation – pin-prick, touch, paraesthesias, or tenderness. Due to the wide variations in neuroanatomy and neurophysiology, taken in isolation these signs are seldom of intrinsic diagnostic value; but taken as a group they commonly indicate the segmental level (and occasionally the specific site) to which musculoskeletal techniques may be profitably applied. Apart from the standard neurological and orthopaedic examination, one particular example demands special comment – saddle anaesthesia (like the sphincter problems that may be revealed in the history) is an indication for instant surgical referral. Details of local examination techniques are to be found in Chapter 2. It is important to stress that, while in the first place these techniques (together with history taking and the chosen therapeutic measures) add appreciably to the doctor's initial consultation time, in the long term they are likely to reduce his work load by reducing the overall number of patient visits (8). Many of these patients go back to work, having no further need of medical assistance.

The danger signals are clearly set out in the report of the CSAG (31) (see Chapter 6). Suffice it to say here that they are crucial to the avoidance of disasters, nearly all of which stem from ignorance or disregard of them. It is not vertebral manipulation that is dangerous, but rather its employment on a patient in whom there exists a contraindication to its use. It is for this reason that we include a list of major contraindications in our data recording sheet as an ever-present reminder to the busy practitioner.

When it comes to therapeutic techniques, the doctor will need to have some choice at each region. The choice depends on the patient's physique, size, and degree of relaxation, the doctor's facilities and the techniques he or she finds easiest to employ. Burn and I recommend teaching physicians two sitting techniques each for the cervical, thoracic, and lumbar regions, two lying techniques for each region, and one standing technique for the thoracic spine, so that each practitioner may make his or her own choices. In practice, the great majority of doctors make use of the techniques they find themselves most comfortable with, seldom using more than four or five manipulative techniques on a daily basis. Using techniques with which they are most comfortable has the advantage of enabling doctors to be better relaxed at the time of manipulation, which adds to the efficacy of their therapy. To this may be added a small range of simple injections.

Doctors must always be on their guard against the nonsense diagnoses that abound. I have already mentioned some. When necessary, they must explain to the patient why some diagnoses are scientifically unacceptable, in terms the patient can understand. Every good consultation has an educational component. Doctors must press the point that lack of a proven diagnosis is not an automatic disadvantage, so long as they recognise and comply with the contraindications to manipulation or simple injections. The same degree of honesty must extend to prognosis. Prediction of result of any musculoskeletal therapy is not supportable (31). Doctors must say so, and must reassure the patient that this does not matter; they must abandon their first choice of therapy if it has not afforded substantial improvement in three sessions. This is honest, practical empiricism, acceptable whenever the contraindications have been excluded. The practice, not uncommon among chiropractors, of prescribing a long series of treatments (33) is quite indefensible. Indeed it is common for vertebral manipulation to dispel the problem in one session (in one uncontrolled series of 1037 patients over 52% in the neck and 23% in the lumbar spine), and very common in three sessions (in the same series over 83% in the neck and 66% in the lumbar spine) (8).

In the U.K. (particularly within the National Health Service), doctors have a number of choices as to how they deal with these cases; the relative costs of these choices vary widely. They may prescribe an analgesic, which will involve most patients in an ever-increasing prescription fee, the taxpayer bearing the brunt of the actual cost, private patients paying all, or passing on the cost to one of the private health insurance companies. They may prescribe bed rest, which prevents the patient from working. They may refer the patient to a physiotherapist, an osteopath, or a chiropractor, either within the practice or without; this costs the practice the appropriate professional fees. They may refer the patient to the hospital, probably involving a long wait. In the case of private patients, either the patient or the insurance company pays. Many years ago the medical director of one of the insurance companies told me that his company was paying £24,000,000 per annum with respect to spinal pain (4). The matter of cost is considered more fully in Chapter 5.

But doctors have a further option: they may deal with most of these patients themselves. This involves the initial cost of learning, which takes the purchase of one manual (5) and three $1^1/_2$-day courses, spread over a year. To offer courses of 300 hours per annum is wholly unnecessary, makes attendance extremely difficult, and is likely to prove confusing. The secondary cost is at first spending more time on these cases, the latter soon reversing itself in becoming a positive gain, due to seeing such patients less often for follow-up. Not only is the practice better off financially, the patient is likely to be relieved sooner (at little cost, and returning to work much sooner), hospital waiting lists (inpatient and outpatient) are likely to be reduced, private insurers are likely to find a sharp fall in their expenditure, and the long-suffering taxpayer will be called upon for less. The Minister of Health may even find something deserving on which to spend the money so saved.

All in all, this seems like good business. But still overall acceptance eludes us. Is it too much to suggest that the general practitioner might actively seek more effective preparation for so important a part of his work? But how?

Chapter 5
The Economics of Musculoskeletal Medicine

I have already referred to the costs of musculoskeletal medicine to patients – or rather the costs of their having a problem in this area. Within the National Health Service (NHS) these costs are prescription charges and loss of earnings. Outside the NHS, in addition to loss of earnings, they involve the full cost of all drugs, plus fees paid to bone setters, physiotherapists, osteopaths, chiropractors, herbalists, acupuncturists, and the few doctors of varying persuasions who have chosen to work outside the NHS. Fees vary widely, but may be substantial, at times quite high. Some of these costs may be recoverable from private health insurance sources, in which case patients have already paid their whack! Some sufferers will be persuaded to purchase specially designed beds, pillows, and chairs (some of dubious efficacy), in addition to the basic costs outlined. These may add up to considerable sums – and a leaking water bed may ruin the ceiling of the room below!

It is difficult to estimate the cost to the NHS. In part this is due to the fact that musculoskeletal problems are not universally recognised at onset, so that the patient may languish for a considerable time in the "wrong" department, and in part to the complexity of both general practice and hospital financing. If it is true that over 90% of these patients first present with these problems in general practice (3), and that only a very small proportion of these patients need to be referred to hospital, the greatest of these costs is likely to be pharmaceutical. It is generally accepted that, in the United Kingdom, the "average" patient sees the general practitioner between five and six times a year. On the basis of a population approaching 60 million, even at the lower figure of five visits this means 300 million visits in toto. Again at the lower estimate of 20% of these being in respect of musculoskeletal problems, this gives a total of 60 million, which makes for an awful lot of pills and potions. When hospitalisation, tests, medical and nursing care, bed occupancy, and operating room use are added, the costs per patient soar. What a blessing that hospital referrals need to be only relatively few. This could so easily become a reality, if only the medical profession were to take on these problems as a part of orthodox care.

It is politically easy to speak of the cost of musculoskeletal problems to the NHS. It is very difficult to make anything like an accurate estimate. Of course, the most important thing to remember is that the NHS pays for nothing. It is the patient/tax-payer who foots the bill for the entire NHS, as it is for private care. It is pertinent to ask what relationship musculoskeletal medical costs bear to the overall aggregate clinical costs, as well as to the hideous administrative costs of the NHS. My strong impression is that today the latter by far exceed the former. While this is but an impression, two illustrations may indicate the size of the problem. In 1913 the administrative staff of the Samaritan Hospital, in the Marylebone Road, in London, numbered just one – and he was pretty grossly overworked. In 1948, in the same building, with the same number of beds (if with a somewhat increased patient turnover) the administrative staff numbered 60! In 1975, when I retired from the NHS, the clerk of the local executive council told me that, in substantial measure to look after the administrative affairs of about 400 doctors, dentists, and pharmacists (paying them once per month, but with no handling of drug pricing), he had a staff numbering 50. One administrator to pay eight people once a month!

The cost to the doctor has already been mentioned, and in this instance I refer largely to family doctors. The cost depends on the form of their contract (ever liable to change) and on the availability of suitably trained ancillary staff, either within the practice or nearby, as well as on their hospital referral rate. But if 57,000 doctors are seeing 60 million musculoskeletal problems a year, the figure must be large indeed, something on the order of 20 per doctor per week. Any sort of referral seems likely to cost the practice a lot of money, regardless of the minutiae of the doctor's contract. The sensible, cost-effective answer for general practitioners must be to deal with most of these cases themselves.

I have already commented on the fact that one of the major health insurers was some years ago spending £24 million per annum on these problems (4). This was by no means the largest company, and the figure is nearly ten years out of date. This is a tiny fraction of the overall cost to the taxpayer, as relatively few patients can afford private insurance. No wonder the politicians are worried about the situation. Clearly, something needs to be done about it. What might happen to these escalating costs, if a substantial number of family doctors dealt with the great majority of these cases within their own practices, earning modest fees in return for saving a huge sum? But how could it be done? Here the medical educators might well be on their guard at the prospect of loading their curricula with still another subject.

But what about the general practitioner? Not yet another subject to study! Not yet more time to be found away from the practice! Not further money to be spent on the process of learning! Yes, precisely that. The government positively encourages postgraduate study, in so doing forcing the taxpayer to subsidise it indirectly. I have already stated that it is possible for the doctor to employ musculoskeletal therapies in safety, with substantial expectation of considerable success in three $1^{1}/_{2}$-day courses. This is only in part true! It can be achieved so quickly after reading and thoroughly digesting a suitable manual (5) and covering the appropriate fees for the courses (see Chapter 6).

So much for the added costs. What are the savings to be expected? Supposing that in a four-person practice one doctor were to attend one of these courses and then take over the musculoskeletal work of the practice. Initially he or she would see about 80 of these patients per week, instead of his or her one-fourth share – 20. But in a very short time the doctor would find that this figure falls considerably, as his or her individual success rate would reduce the overall practice work load dramatically by lowering the number of follow-up attendances. This decline would be cumulative and would commence almost immediately, as the courses are designed so as to permit the employment of vertebral manipulation and simple injections on one region of the spine the day after the doctor finishes the first short course of the series. Within the year he or she would be able to take full advantage of these techniques at any segmental level. The practice would find its spending on referral to ancillaries and to the hospital plummeting; in rural practices, spending on analgesics and antiinflammatory drugs would fall as well.

Of course, it would make a much stronger case if the number of new musculoskeletal patients seen per week in the practice were known, if the average number of return visits were known (before and after inclusion of these techniques), and if the average success rate were known. If vertebral manipulation costs no more than a few minutes' time, an injection in addition costs one syringe, one needle, and a small sum for local anaesthetic, with or without steroid, the cost-effectiveness must be good. Clearly this is good business for the doctors. And it should be remembered that the same costs may eventually be incurred in the hospital, in addition to the cost of referral on top of the cost of tests.

The savings for patients would be as dramatic. First, they would be likely to find a big decrease in their absences from work, with lessening of the risk of their problem becoming chronic, and a considerable decrease in prescription charges, quite apart from the likely early decrease in pain. Second, they would find a reduction in waiting time for a hospital appointment, if referral were found necessary. Third, they would have less occasion to pay private practitioners of any persuasion for treatment and, if the size of the problem is as big as I have indicated, a reduction of their need to rely on private health insurance. It seems highly likely that patients would approve such a move.

The really big savings would come for taxpayers. Even without slimming down the currently grossly top-heavy NHS administration, they would save many millions of pounds per annum. They would surely welcome such a move. A lot of people stand to save a great deal of money through the re-adoption of musculoskeletal medicine by the medical establishment and its concentration in primary care. It is a question of simple logic: if primary care takes on the major part of the burden of musculoskeletal problems, this is likely to commonly permit earlier return to work. It is also likely to reduce referral to hospital for costly tests and even more costly hospitalisation. Whatever the actual savings are shown to be, they may be expected to be more than substantial.

But how? Will this not of itself involve new and as yet unassessed costs? This issue is addressed in Chapters 6 and 15.

Chapter 6
Teaching Musculoskeletal Medicine

The scientific bases of musculoskeletal medicine have been discussed in Chapter 2. Their importance lies chiefly in their being thoroughly understood, including understanding how little we really know, and how we may best safely overcome our shortage of proven facts. Unfortunately for the patient, in spite of the compelling arguments in favour of the subject being regarded as wholly orthodox, and in spite of the fact that it so commonly presents in general practice, provision of suitable teaching facilities remains scant. I am aware of only one university in the United Kingdom where it appears, optionally, in the undergraduate curriculum – the University of Newcastle. I know of only two universities where it is an optional extra in postgraduate teaching of primary care rheumatology – the University of Bath, in collaboration with the Primary Care Rheumatology Society, and the University of Southampton, in association with the British Institute of Musculoskeletal Medicine. Many doctors and patients must regard this dearth of courses as unsatisfactory.

In addition to these programs, there are the London School of Osteopathy (for nonmedical students), the London College of Osteopathic Medicine (exclusively for medically qualified students), and the Anglo-American College of Chiropractic in Bournemouth (open to nonmedical students). Courses for doctors are also offered by the British Institute of Musculoskeletal Medicine. Otherwise, Dr. Loïc Burn and I ran comprehensive courses from 1983 for a good many years, most recently at the West Middlesex University Hospital. It is of further interest that in France, due in great measure to the influence of Dr. Robert Maigne, the elements of musculoskeletal medicine have been included in the medical curricula of at least fourteen universities. Some schools of physiotherapy also teach manipulative techniques.

In Chapter 2 I mentioned the six essentials to rapid learning in this field. Here I shall look more closely at each in turn. First is the epidemiology of pain of vertebral origin. In some countries it is omitted from the curriculum altogether! It is imperative to remember a number of facts. As long ago as 1971 Wiltze (34) showed that there was no direct correlation between back pain and skeletal defect. In 1976 Torgerson and Dotter (35) found no proven correlation between back pain and degenerative changes, except when those changes were really gross. In 1969 Collis and Ponsetti (36) demonstrated no proven correlation between back pain and postural abnormality, unless the latter was gross. In spite of the common belief that patients with these conditions are doomed to progressive, lifelong worsening, this is just not the case, as the incidence of these problems falls substantially after the age of 55, although the degenerative process continues unabated (37). There is some not wholly satisfactory evidence of a causal relationship between back pain and physically heavy work, static work postures, frequent bending and twisting and other forceful movements, repetitive work, and vibration (38–40). There is again some relationship between back pain and genetic factors, such as human leukocyte antigen (HLA) B27 (3). According to Professor Houssemaine DuBoulay, an evolutionary cause is not supported by currently available evidence. Age, gender, and posture are poorly correlated with the incidence of back pain, the latter including differences in leg length (41,42). These are all matters that may be learned by reading the manual by Burn (5), thereby greatly reducing the time necessarily spent on practical courses.

Pain perception and modulation have been considered in Chapter 2 (17), together with the important phenomena of referred pain and referred tenderness (14–16). While the theory may be learned by reading, these twin phenomena claim a greater place in practical teaching, referred tenderness forming a major part of local examination of the spine. While the patient will be clear as to the site of perception of his pain, this may well differ widely from its site of origin, the latter commonly exhibiting tenderness and apparent restriction of movement (by pain, muscle spasm, or both).

The detailed anatomy relating to these problems is important. Again, the more important points have been presented in Chapter 2. Once more they may best be learned from an appropriate manual, prior to attending a practical course, revision and discussion taking up relatively little time. The first item of importance is the course of the vertebral artery above the second cervical level, rendering it possible to occlude one in certain positions, if held for too long. If the other artery is blocked by an atheroma, it is in this way possible to cause irreversible brain damage by cutting off the blood supply to the circle of Willis (24). Clearly this is a strong argument in favour of not testing by pro- longed rotation in extension (a procedure still widely taught), rather relying on a careful history.

The second is the predilection of rheumatoid arthritis for the odontoid process, rendering it all too easy to destroy the spinal cord by direct trauma. The patient (43). Coupled with this is Grisel's syndrome, in which a sore throat in a young child may cause prolonged weakening of the transverse and apical liga- ments of the odontoid process – with similar attendant risks (44). It will be noted that this condition was first described a very long time ago – 1930 – yet few doctors know of it!

The presence of cervical ribs may present a problem, but this is by no means inevitable, the condition appearing quite fre- quently in the asymptomatic patient. Asymmetry of the spinous processes, perfectly normal and most common in the thoracic region, may prove misleading, often giving rise to the insup- portable view that a particular vertebra is rotated in relation to its neighbours (45). Clearly, basing a system of diagnosis on such a finding is unscientific, putting the patient at risk of an unsuit- able treatment being chosen.

The pelvic joints, both the sacroiliac and the symphysis pubis, are the source of further misunderstanding. In spite of some teaching, predominantly that of schools of osteopathy (25), it must be remembered that the sacroiliac joints are the largest in the body, their opposing surfaces deeply and irregularly pitted (with prominences to fit the pits) and supported by the strongest ligaments in the body. These two factors greatly restrict move- ment and thereby reduce the chance of these joints being the source of painful problems by any appreciable degree of malpo- sition. Indeed, it is doubtful whether they do indeed cause pain at all. What needs to be remembered is that pain felt at this site is commonly referred from a distant origin, and that this may be revealed by local examination of the spine. It is, of course, the site of origin of such pain to which therapy should be directed, rather than its site of perception.

The symphysis pubis is a relatively rare site of origin of pain, as it is seldom greatly stressed, apart from in the second stage of labour, where damage may be done by a distracting force on the pubic disc, rather than a compression force as in the case of intervertebral disc damage. Of course, damage may arise from complex accidents, where manipulation would in any case be contraindicated. Indeed, a substantial compression force is diffi- cult to apply to the pubic disc, owing to the relatively minor movement possible at the sacroiliac joints and the rigidity of the pelvic bones. Again, the subjective impression of asymmetry in the level of the pubic bones is of no diagnostic significance.

The relevant pathology has been referred to in earlier chapters in this book, and rheumatoid arthritis and Grisel's syndrome in this chapter. Recent fracture, substantial osteoporosis, and secondary cancers of bone present obvious dangers, as stressed in the Clinical Standards Advisory Group (CSAG) report (31) and other sources already quoted. Out of these emerge the absolute and the relative contraindications for manipulative therapies, of the utmost importance in reading prior to practical courses, and necessarily recapitulated on the courses themselves. It is only by the rigorous adherence to these contraindications that vertebral manipulation is shown to be so safe a therapy (5).

At this point it is worthwhile again mentioning systematised data recording – for three reasons. First, it counters the initial reaction of students that there is a great deal of new material to remember and an awful lot to write down. Far from it. In practice, by the use of a simple system it is possible to record data more quickly than by writing words or personal variations in shorthand, or entering them onto disc in note form; and those data are more rapidly recovered. Second, the inclusion of the important contraindications on the form acts as a reminder in history taking. Third, and perhaps most important of all, such data recording renders possible accurate comparison of data for research purposes. Such a system is to be found in both the course manual (5) and in a book written to promote international coordination of teaching (45). The system is to be found in Chapter 2 of this book.

The basic skills required fall into two categories: diagnostic and therapeutic. At once we face a problem in the use of the word *diagnosis*. As previously reported, it is seldom possible to make a definitive diagnosis in the spine, a view supported by the CSAG report (31). Burn and I favour six basic diagnostic procedures, whereby it is commonly possible to make practical decisions as to how to proceed therapeutically, in particular where to apply any local therapeutic choice, such as manipulation or injection. These six procedures are skin pinching; assessment of paravertebral muscle tone; search for trigger points; segmental sagittal pressure (with the exception of the cervical spine); lateral spinous process pressure, which induces a degree of rotation between adjacent vertebrae (again with the exception of the cervical spine); and a search for zygoapophyseal tenderness. To these are added three pelvic tests. These are illustrated in Chapter 2.

It must be stressed that these are in addition to the standard orthopaedic and neurological examination taught in all medical schools, rather than as an alternative. These are described in the course manual (5), and they should again be described and demonstrated to the class in the practical courses, demonstrated a second time by the instructor on every student, before being practiced by every student. Thus, each student has read about it, heard about it, seen it, felt it performed by an expert, performed it him- or herself, and felt it performed by a novice. Teaching these procedures in this manner necessarily limits the number of students that may be accommodated in each course, which is not a bad thing in a practical setting!

The manual therapeutic techniques are dealt with similarly. In contrast to the osteopathic tendency to teach literally hundreds of techniques, what is found in everyday practice is that experienced practitioners of all persuasions habitually use just a few, perhaps five or six. Because the perceived preferences and the physical facilities available vary so widely from practice to practice, it seems sensible to teach two sitting techniques and two supine techniques for the cervical spine, applicable to different spinal levels. Similarly, two sitting techniques and one supine and one prone technique are sufficient for the thoracic spine, with the addition of one standing technique (including a number of variations). Again, the lumbar spine teaching requires two sitting and two lying techniques.

It is wise to teach all these techniques in three stages. The first stage is setting up each in turn, in rotation with or without flexion or extension. The second stage is taking up the slack, to the limit of comfort of the patient. The third stage should not actually be performed in the courses, except in the case of a student with a suitable history and appropriate local signs and in the absence of contraindications. It is the employment of a thrust, which is an exacerbation of all the elements of positioning and taking up the slack, performed with maximal speed and minimal amplitude. It is most important that any thrust be made from the position of the slack having been taken up, without relaxing the second stage. In practice, the third stage must be abandoned in the case of the patient complaining of increased pain on taking up the slack.

The reason for this approach is that it offers students alternatives, recognising that they might be working in different types of facilities. For example, if there is not enough space in a consulting room to have a free-standing couch, sitting techniques are clearly worth considering. On the other hand, with a free-standing couch, lying techniques offer the advantage that it is easier for the patient to relax, an important factor contributing to both more accurate assessment and the greater likelihood of successful vertebral manipulation. It is important to stress that, due to anatomical differences among manipulators (including size, strength, and gender) as well as the physical and emotional differences between patients, the particular technique chosen is very much an individual matter. In practice each manipulator develops his own techniques within the basic parameters of safety and likely efficacy.

In addition to these manual techniques a series of local injections should be taught. These include peripheral nerve block, injection of trigger points and of attachment tissues, in the vicinity of posterior vertebral joints, as well as caudal epidurals, the latter to be used only where adequate resuscitation facilities exist on site. In this last case, it is stressed that there is no need to attempt to enter the posterior joints; without radiological control it is virtually impossible, and from a practical point of view it is quite unnecessary. In view of the overlap of spinal innervation, it is worthwhile also injecting the levels immediately above and below, and all that is required after the injection is a vigorous rub to disperse the local anaesthetic in the vicinity – at the same time affording further mechanoceptor stimulation! It is stressed that the injection techniques should be taught without penetrating the skin (particularly caudal epidurals) using skin marking on students by ballpoint pen. In the absence of patients on courses, it is not acceptable to perform actual injections, but students must feel free to discuss their deployment with their local consultants prior to actually using them in practice, if they so wish.

With a series of three practical courses, one primarily devoted to the neck, one to the thorax, and one to the lumbar spine, in each course the work of the other two regions should be revised. Students should be strongly urged to practice only what they have learned in depth, but they have the advantage of seeing the techniques for the other regions and, of course, they automatically revise what they have already learned in previous courses, and they must feel free to discuss any problems they may have encountered. Further, it does not matter at which point they start the courses, as long as they have read and absorbed the manual thoroughly. This makes it easier for them to coordinate the courses with their practice commitments.

Approached in this way, past results have proved most encouraging. The great majority of students return to their practices actively seeking suitable patients. Many are astonished at the initial results of their manipulative efforts. Numerous course assessments have been very encouraging, especially from consultant and trainee rheumatologists (commonly over 90% approval in all aspects of the courses). A number of students have returned for refresher courses 1 or 2 years after their introductory courses. Perhaps the most important feature of such teaching, apart from stressing safety, is that there is nothing difficult about it. If you can ride a bicycle and play Ping-Pong, you already have the neuromuscular coordination to master the manual techniques very rapidly. There is no virtue in teaching dozens of techniques. The claim that this is necessitated by specific diagnoses demanding specific techniques is just not valid.

Today there exists a strong demand for evidence of the efficacy of vertebral manipulation. This is a perfectly reasonable attitude. However, satisfaction of this demand presents several difficulties. The first is that, as has been mentioned earlier, a definitive diagnosis, other than the blanket diagnosis of simple back pain (or pain of vertebral origin) is commonly impossible, largely due to the known asymmetry of the vertebrae and to the complexity and flexibility of the neuromuscular control systems. Simple back pain is far from specific, so diagnosis is most often presumptive. Identical conditions are commonly labeled differently by students of the different schools. The inevitable result of this must be that researchers can seldom be sure that they are comparing like with like. Nevertheless, three studies are worth mentioning.

A review of 35 randomised clinical trials showed poor-quality trial design or conduct in the majority, with but four deemed adequate; of these, one showed definite benefit from manipulation, one showed no benefit, and two showed some improvement only (46). A trial with a year's follow-up, comparing manipulation with (unspecified) physiotherapy, general practice management, and placebo showed a clear advantage for manipulation (47). (It is well to bear in mind that there is no such thing as a placebo manipulation, as every physical contact with the patient must result in some degree of mechanoceptor stimulation.) A large-scale trial comparing chiropractic with hospital outpatient treatment came down firmly in favour of manipulation (48).

A second concern is that of safety. I have already pointed out that the great majority of dangers may be avoided by strict adherence to the contraindications to vertebral manipulation. One review worth quoting covered 135 cases of severe complication; 50% were in the cervical spine, and 26 of the total cases were due to frank misdiagnosis. A further finding of interest was that the problems occurred more often when performed with the patient under general anaesthesia (49). The latter finding accords with our teaching on the subject; with the patient under general anaesthesia the doctor is inevitably denied the most important of all the contraindications – the patient's report of increased pain on setting it up or taking up the slack. Yet the practice persists in some quarters.

So much for the nuts and bolts of teaching in this field. The question of implementation, together with its costs and savings, is addressed in Chapter 15.

Chapter 7
Headache and Migraine

Head pain is a very common symptom. It may be unilateral, bilateral, occipital, vertical, frontal, parietal, or facial, each with a widely varying intensity. Its severity is commonly affected by bright light, noise, anxiety, or depression. It may be initiated by trauma to the head or neck, primary or secondary tumours of the brain, feverish illnesses, glaucoma, frontal sinusitis, maxillary antritis, or dental sepsis. Of course, musculoskeletal medicine has no place in the management of any of these conditions, other than a small proportion of the traumatic ones. Other than dental therapy or antibiotics, where appropriate, by far the commonest treatments on offer are the wide variety of analgesics, allopathic or homeopathic, available with or without prescription. At times headache is used to attract attention or to avoid unwanted activities, which demands a quite different approach (21). On the other hand, although not widely enough appreciated, headache commonly arises in the cervical spine.

If unilateral, headache is not infrequently labeled migraine, even in the absence of the other factors implicated in true migraine, rather than as an example of pain of vertebral origin (PVO). This is a pity, as it may lead to persistence with inappropriate therapy and thereby delay in dealing with the actual cause of pain. It appears likely that more than 50% of unilateral head pain is not true migraine. Differentiation between the two relies on both history and local examination of the head and neck. The presence of unilateral local physical signs suggests a mechanical cause, in which case vertebral manipulation has to be considered – in the absence of contraindications. If this works, a substantial number of investigations and therapies may be avoided, increasing cost-effectiveness as well as ridding the patient of an unpleasant symptom earlier. If it does not work, an alternative therapy must be sought, or referral may be indicated.

Headache may be accompanied by vertigo, pallor, sweating, nausea, or tinnitus (50). These symptoms need to be pursued. In particular it must be remembered that the patient with tinnitus is commonly referred to an ear, nose, and throat (ENT) or neurological department. If no cause is found, the patient is quite likely to be labeled a malingerer, or the tinnitus or other symptoms may be dismissed as being of psychological origin. Once more, local examination of the head and neck may reveal an asymmetrical pattern of physical signs, indicating cervical manipulation as the therapy of choice.

On one occasion I manipulated a man's neck for unilateral vertical headache (in the presence of abnormal local physical signs and in the absence of contraindications), only to be told I had cured his long-standing tinnitus, the existence of which I was blissfully unaware of! After discussing this with a very experienced colleague, the late Dr. Maxwell Robertson, I was delighted to receive detailed clinical notes of several similar cases that he had found, and thereafter made a practice of questioning all patients with head or neck symptoms as to whether or not they had concomitant tinnitus. This was rewarded by success in treating by cervical manipulation a number of cases of known tinnitus. If it works, this is the quickest and cheapest therapeutic option; if it does not, a change of tactic, probably involving referral, is indicated.

I have already said that vertigo may accompany headache (51). If it is initiated by the patient looking up and to one side, perhaps to a high shelf, it is a contraindication to manipulation, as previously described; it may indicate atheromatous blockage of one vertebral artery. If no cause is apparent, it is again well worthwhile examining the head and neck for asymmetry of local physical signs. In the absence of contraindications, cervical manipulation should be considered at an early stage – on the presumptive diagnosis of cervical posterior joint dysfunction – preferably as the first therapeutic choice. An unpredictable proportion of patients respond well to this approach. Even in the absence of headache, it is sensible to perform a local examination of the head and cervical spine in those complaining of vertigo, considering local vertebral action when asymmetry of signs is revealed. Indeed, local examination of the whole spine is recommended as a routine, as this alerts the doctor to the possibility of the patient's symptoms being of musculoskeletal origin – at any level, and however remote the abnormal signs may be from the perceived site of pain. Contrary to the belief of some, this is not an unacceptably time-consuming practice, and it certainly commonly pays dividends in directing attention to a therapy that is quite likely to prove helpful and carries few risks to the patient.

Visual symptoms are well known to accompany true migraine, but they may also occur in the absence of head pain. Two of the latter are worth mentioning. In a normal state, with the eyes closed, vitreous floaters may slowly wander downward, especially after looking upward. In other circumstances, particularly in the presence of unsuspected cervical spine problems, they may deviate slowly to one side, and then suddenly flick sideways in the other direction. Again in the presence of cervical problems, rapid change of posture (like lying down after standing or sitting) with the eyes open may provoke apparent movement in whatever is being observed, slowly in one direction and rapidly in the other. In the presence of asymmetry of local physical signs in the neck and in the absence of contraindications, both of these phenomena are often eliminated by cervical manipulation. Once more, the presumptive diagnosis is upper cervical posterior joint dysfunction. I have no data regarding success rates but, in the absence of contraindication to manipulation, I have seen no adverse effects. There is, of course, no guarantee of success.

It is not uncommon for patients to fail to mention some of these symptoms. History taking must be adjusted to take this into consideration. I know of one patient who for years periodically assured her doctor that her frontal sinusitis had flared up again. He believed her. It was only after a major detachment of one retina, resulting in almost total blindness in one eye, that her underlying chronic glaucoma was discovered! But her nonsinusitis could just as likely have been referred pain from the region of one of her upper cervical posterior joints. For this reason it is imperative to ask pertinent questions in taking a history; of course, it takes a little longer than skimping things and relying on the patient to volunteer all the necessary information, but it is time well spent. Accepting the patient's diagnosis too readily is seen to be a grave mistake.

Although posture has never been adequately identified as an epidemiological cause of spinal pain (except in extreme cases), it is important to note it, in case of posttherapeutic change. Basic movements should also be included, noting differences in range of flexion, extension, side bending, and rotation, and at the same time noting which movements provoke exacerbation of the patient's pain. Graphical recording of results saves time and affords rapid recall at subsequent visits. An acceptably comprehensive yet adequate example of this is to be found in Chapter 2. Such recall may be similarly achieved with suitable software design in the event of records being computerized. It is vital to regard local examination, at all segmental levels, as an addition to orthopaedic or neurological examination – never as a substitute.

The local physical signs to be sought were described in Chapter 2. In essence, what one is seeking is differences between left and right in each test. It is the sum of findings that commonly indicates the segmental level and the side to which one may best direct one's chosen therapy. It is important to remember that it does not identify a formal diagnosis.

The first local test is to seek tenderness on pinching a roll of skin and subcutaneous tissue (mainly posteriorly, but also to some degree anteriorly), at serial symmetrical levels on the two sides. Because of the phenomenon of referred tenderness, it is necessary to include the eyebrows and the edges of the mandibles, as well as the anterior neck and upper thorax. Again, it is essential first to ask the patient to report if he feels any difference between the two sides; second, to pinch with the same degree of vigour on each side; and third, to record the segmental levels at which differences are reported. It is interesting that, in the event of differences in tenderness being reported, it is not uncommon to find differences in thickness of the skinfold raised by closely similar degrees of pinching – and for this difference to disappear immediately on resolution of the patient's symptoms, thus eliminating the perhaps remote possibility of this being due to local oedema. No explanation is offered for this phenomenon – it is simply an observation that may have significance.

Just as in the acute abdomen (taken for granted by every doctor), muscle guarding is commonly found in the paravertebral muscles of the neck, usually unilaterally, and at any segmental level. Muscle tone on either side must be compared at successive levels, by the application of light pressure at each site. While this is a subjective impression only, what matters is the discovery of differences between the two sides. Positive findings in this test must be recorded.

Much has been written about trigger points (52). In the case of head pain, these may again be identified by pressure applied in symmetrical pattern. They may be found at any level in the neck, but particularly in the trapezii and along the medial margins of the scapulae. Lower down such findings are more common, particularly along the crests of the ilea. Again, it is necessary to instruct the patient to report tenderness provoked by more or less random finger pressure on the two sides, and for this to be recorded. There is a strong temptation to regard these as examples of referred tenderness.

While important elsewhere, the segmental sagittal pressure test, applying a fore-and-aft sliding force to each vertebra in turn, is inapplicable in the neck, in view of the shortness of the spinous processes of the cervical vertebrae making it impossible to define them accurately enough. This will be discussed for lower regions.

In the same way, the lateral spinous process pressure test, applying a rotational force to each vertebra in relation to its neighbours, is inapplicable in the neck and will be discussed for lower regions.

Tenderness directly over the posterior vertebral joints is an important local sign. Once again it is necessary to instruct the patient to report any differences in tenderness between left and right, while pressing with equal force on either side. In the neck it is best performed with the patient supine, as in this position greater muscular relaxation may be expected, so that palpation is rendered easier. The importance of a positive finding lies in it being the most accurate indicator as to where the doctor should direct his chosen therapy – be it vertebral manipulation or injection. If the latter option is taken, it should be remembered that there is no need to enter the joint, and in the absence of radiological control this is virtually impossible. However, in view of the overlap in nerve supply, both up and down, it is worthwhile injecting also the regions of the posterior vertebral joints immediately above and below. This is applicable throughout the length of the spine, with the exception of the first cervical level, where injection should be strictly avoided as being potentially dangerous, in view of the tortuous course of the vertebral artery. This is illustrated in Chapter 2. Fuller details of these techniques are to be found in the appropriate course manual (5).

Contraindications to vertebral manipulation fall into two groups: absolute and relative. Perhaps of prime importance in the former group is the rheumatoid neck (43). The reason for this is that rheumatoid weakening of the transverse ligament of the odontoid process permits its dislocation, with attendant serious risk to life by pressure on the spinal cord. The rheumatoid odontoid process may also be fractured by vigorous manipulation. This is illustrated in Chapter 2. As previously noted, vigorous procedures are themselves contraindicated, as these provide no therapeutic advantage over gentle ones, as well as being unkind to the patient.

Grisel's syndrome is a condition in which a child with an upper respiratory infection may suffer hypermobility of the upper cervical spine, due to ligamentous laxity, carrying similar risks to the rheumatoid neck (43). It is important to remember

that such hypermobility may persist for some weeks after resolution of the infection. It is improbable that this vital history will
be volunteered by the patient; it must be sought.

Cervical myelopathy, in which the vascular supply to the
spinal cord is already poor, is an absolute contraindication. The
same applies to the thoracic region and to the lumbar spine –
hence the importance of saddle anaesthesia and sphincter disorders, to be discussed later in this book.

The relative contraindications to cervical vertebral manipulation are three. If all movements or attempted movements cause
pain, then therapies other than manipulation should be given a
chance. For the general practitioner, these include oral analgesics, gentle traction, local anaesthetic injection, transcutaneous electrical nerve stimulation (TENS), and acupuncture.

If the spine is grossly stiff, the same considerations apply,
although it is impossible to know how flexible the patient was
before the onset of symptoms.

When it comes to manipulative techniques, if on "taking up
the slack"[1] the patient complains of an appreciable increase in
pain, the particular manoeuvre should not be pursued. This latter
is probably the most frequently useful contraindication, as vertebral manipulation should always be gentle, and the use of too
great a force is unkind, unnecessary, and potentially harmful. *If
it hurts, do not do it!* Of course, this raises serious doubts as to
the acceptability of vertebral manipulation under general anaesthesia, as patients are in no position to complain of their increase
of pain. It is potentially extremely dangerous. This applies to the
whole length of the spine.

Psychological factors have already been touched upon (21).
Perhaps the commonest psychological cause of headache is
worry. The sources for that worry are legion. Such a situation
may prove hard to define. Clearly, history is all-important, but it
must be remembered that patients do not always volunteer their
anxiety, so it is wise to enquire about it. Of course, trauma is
obvious to all, but in the absence of trauma, fear of what unex-
plained headache may presage is important. If fear enters into
the causation of the pain, it must be included in what is treated
by explanation of the problem in terms the patient can understand. Vertebral manipulation is unlikely to alleviate depression
or fear!

---

[1]"Taking up the slack" is the process of continuing a movement or
complex of movements to the limit of the comfort of the patient, mandatory prior to any vertebral manipulation.

I do not intend to describe specific therapeutic techniques. As made clear in Chapter 6, reading an appropriate manual as a precursor to attending practical courses is mandatory in acquiring competence and assuring safety.

But it is worthwhile considering the likely results that may be expected in nonmigrainous headache. An asymmetrical pattern of the local physical signs described earlier in this chapter is likely to present. In the absence of contraindications, cervical manipulation is quite likely to eliminate the headache within three sessions, and often in one. If it has not, then other therapies should be considered. I have already cited a series of 364 unselected patients with cervical problems treated in this way in whom 51% were pain free after one treatment, a further 21.2% after a second treatment, and another 10.7% after a third. Clearly, the prescription of a lengthy series of treatments at first consultation is clinically and morally insupportable, yet it is quite commonly practiced, particularly by chiropractors.

Chapter 8
Neck Pain

Onset of pain in the neck may be sudden, as in direct trauma to the head or neck (accidental or by design), or whiplash injury (karate or motor vehicle accident). Or it may be insidious, as in a high proportion of cases. In the sudden-onset group the preferred management is usually clear, except in the very low degree whiplash injury where, after rigorous assessment, it may prove useful to employ light cervical traction or very gentle manipulation. The insidious-onset group demands the same degree of rigour in assessment, in history taking, in main-line orthopaedic and neurological examination, and in local examination. Chronic whiplash injury that has not responded to other treatments may be considered for traction or vertebral manipulation – in the presence of abnormal local signs and in the absence of contraindications.

Although mostly intermittent or at least variable in severity, some patients present with constant pain. The latter are more likely to have a systemic cause for their pain, including rheumatoid arthritis, gross degenerative changes, severe hypertension, bony metastases, myeloma, or the pain sometimes persisting after polymyalgia rheumatica. Apart from those cases due to metastases or hypertension, these chronic cases are usually best referred to multidisciplinary pain clinics. As with headache, some cases seem to be related to work posture, particularly for those working with computers. In this event, it may prove beneficial and a lot less expensive to experiment with screen, keyboard, and seat heights before referral to the pain clinic. The same considerations apply to pianists.

Pain on movement in one direction or another is common, frequently resulting in restriction of range in the painful direction. Pain on resisted movement is also common, although I refer to this as pain on obstructed movement. Movement on testing should be eliminated as much as possible, not just challenged. Causes to be considered are many, including perhaps lesser degrees of those mentioned in the preceding paragraph. Pain perception being so very much an individual matter, it is impossible to measure, but it is possible to compare the comfortable range of movement in opposite directions – to the left and right in side bending, rotation, and (with less accuracy) between flexion and extension, each with and without obstruction to movement.

It must be remembered that spinal movements at all segmental levels are commonly asymmetrical in range in the absence of symptoms. In the concomitant absence of abnormal local signs, it is reasonable to regard such asymmetry as normal for the individual. This advice is intimately related to the fact that no vertebra is perfectly symmetrical in form, and that no two vertebrae are precisely similar, in which case perfect symmetry of movement in the asymptomatic would of course be surprising. Returning to the neck, the proposal still sometimes put forward that pain-free patients should be able to put their ears on their shoulders is both ludicrous and potentially dangerous. Nonetheless, it is still put forward from time to time.

It is important to remember that pain of vertebral origin may be referred both upward and downward. Pain referred upward was discussed in the previous chapter. Downward referral may give rise to pain in the trapezii, the shoulders, the arms, and the interscapular region. Less commonly it may be referred anteriorly to the chest, at times mimicking pain of cardiac origin, although, as will be discussed in Chapter 10, the commoner origin for such pain is from around the fourth thoracic segmental level (16). In view of the fact that pain fibres commonly overlap by several segments, both within the spinal cord and without, it is not surprising that the anterior branches of segmental nerves are at times involved in this way.

With the exception of trauma, such as whiplash injury, the history is most commonly of insidious onset of pain. Postural causes have to be considered, particularly in office workers, and suitable avoiding action taken where indicated. Pillow height may be important, especially in the elderly, although this is unlikely to emerge from the history, unless specific enquiry is made. Such enquiry therefore should be routine.

Local examination is as described in the previous chapter, with the exception of excluding skin pinching at the eyebrow and mandible. They are illustrated in Chapter 2. The discovery of asymmetrical local signs in the absence of contraindications suggests the presumptive diagnosis of simple spinal pain and the tentative deployment of vertebral manipulation as the therapy of preference, with injection as the immediate backup.

Contraindications to vertebral manipulation are as already described. Assiduous data recording is again vital, a standard format reducing the time taken to enter data as well as the time to recall them (see Chapter 2). In view of the very common impossibility of making a valid, definitive diagnosis, the ability to review changes in findings on local examination is of paramount importance.

Therapeutic techniques should never be learned from a text alone. As stressed in Chapter 6, they should be read, described, demonstrated, and practiced under close supervision, before being employed on patients. In practice they will be modified to suit both the manipulator and the patient, and further slight modification of all techniques will be made with experience. Every manipulator makes a personal choice from the techniques taught, and this choice depends at least in part on practice circumstances. This is of no consequence, so long as assessment is thorough, data recording is meticulous and the contraindications are rigidly adhered to. As previous stated, this is the rationale for teaching two sitting and two lying techniques for the cervical spine, in the full expectation that three of the four will be discarded by most students – though not the same three!

Traction has to be considered in those patients for whom manipulation is contraindicated, particularly in the elderly, who may suffer from undiagnosed osteoporosis, but it remains unlikely that suitably gentle vertebral manipulation will damage relatively fragile bone, in the absence of a compression force. No such compression is to be found in the techniques taught. If traction is employed, it may be done either in the consulting room or in the patient's home. In either case it should be remembered that the head weighs about 14 pounds, so to produce similar results the traction applied needs to be appreciably more if the patient is standing or sitting rather than lying down. A ten-pound pull on the standing or sitting patient does not apply any degree of traction at all; it does not even take off the compression force due to head weight. The patient does more by putting his head on his pillow! Of some interest is the availability of the DIY (do it yourself) traction apparatus, suitable for use in these conditions (Figs. 8.1 and 8.2).

The apparatus is hung from a fixed point, which must be secure. The spreader frame may be even simpler than that illustrated, in that it needs to have only two hooks that are set a distance apart. From this is hung the head harness. This is very simple and fits any head. For domiciliary use, it is best to adjust the level of the harness to that which permits its fitting with the

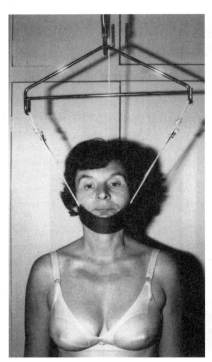 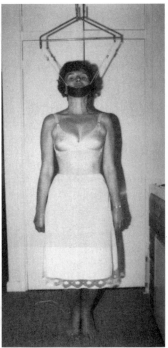

FIGURE 8.1. DIY cervical traction apparatus. (From Paterson JK, Burn L. *An Introduction to Medical Manipulation*. Lancaster, England: MTP Press, 1985, p. 180.)

patient standing comfortably. The two slings of the harness are placed at the chin and the occiput, a gentle wriggle adjusting them to suit the individual shape of the head. Traction – up to any strength of pull acceptable to the patient – is applied by the patient's gently sagging at the knee, reducing the weight placed on the feet. The pull thus applied may be maintained as long as it is comfortable. When the patient has had enough, he or she just stands up. This may be repeated several times per session, and it is reasonable to use this apparatus several times a day, when the patient finds it convenient.

The use of collars should be viewed with circumspection. Although they act chiefly to remind patients of their problem, they do not markedly restrict movement. But they do inevitably alter the cervical reflexes, rendering the wearer at substantial risk

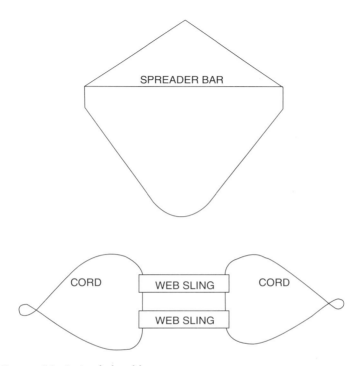

FIGURE 8.2. A simple head harness.

in activities like driving a car (24). Patients' control of their arms and legs may be impaired. The latter fact is not widely enough appreciated. Collars are of little or no proven therapeutic value, yet they are commonly prescribed.

Results of cervical manipulation, as reported in relation to head pain, are very encouraging. As previously reported, in an unselected series of 364 cases with cervical problems, 51.9% were pain free in one session, 22.2% more in two sessions, and a further 10.7% in three sessions (8), including patients with cervical signs accompanying head symptoms.

Chapter 9
Shoulder and Arm Pain

Shoulder pain may arise locally, quite commonly including fractures, various forms of arthritis, and sprains of any of the supporting ligaments. On the other hand, identical pain may arise remote from the site of pain, in the cervical or upper thoracic spine. Fractures should be easy to identify. The pain of acute arthritis is usually constant, with exacerbation on attempted movement. Rheumatoid arthritis is usually easy to identify, as is degenerative arthrosis, and both are likely to involve more than one joint, although perhaps not at the onset of symptoms. Polymyalgia rheumatica may cause some diagnostic difficulty, as, contrary to some teaching, the erythrocyte sedimentation rate (ESR) is not invariably raised. Ligamentous sprains are suggested from the history and confirmed by adequate examination. In this case exacerbation of pain is commonly found on certain movements only, on stretching joint capsules and their supporting ligaments. One of the commonest conditions in this region is anterior capsulitis. *Frozen shoulder* is a term I prefer not to use, except to imply the chronicity of shoulder pain related to unsuccessful or inappropriate treatment.

Rheumatoid arthritis and polymyalgia rheumatica are best treated in the orthodox manner, primarily with nonsteroidal anti-inflammatory drugs. Nonrheumatoid arthritis may be treated with analgesics and, in the case of sepsis being identified, an appropriate antibiotic. Degenerative arthrosis may be severe enough to warrant intraarticular injection of local anaesthetic and steroid; my preference is to take the posterior approach, simply because I find it more easy to enter the joint. Intraarticular opioids or α_2-adrenergic agonists may also be considered, although some general practitioners regard them as belonging to the specialist domain. They are used in addition to analgesics, if need be.

Ligamentous strains are best dealt with by local anaesthetic injection at the site of pain, with or without added steroids, although the more severe or chronic cases may warrant intraarticular injection. Anterior capsular pain is best treated by local anaesthetic and steroid injection. However, in the event of asymmetry of local signs being found in the lower cervical and upper thoracic spine, and in the absence of contraindications, cervicothoracic manipulation is quite likely to prove effective and should be considered as the treatment of first choice because it is quick to perform, noninvasive, inexpensive, and safe. But first these signs must be sought! X-ray or other scanning is of course indicated in case of doubt.

Tennis elbow is a well-known condition in which the tendon insertions into the lateral epicondyle of the humerus are overstressed. Orthodox therapy is rest, analgesics, or local anaesthetic and steroid injection; rarely is surgical intervention required. It is not widely enough appreciated that pain and tenderness at this site may also be referred from the lower cervical and upper thoracic spine. It is therefore imperative to perform local examination of the spine before embarking on any invasive therapy. This is well illustrated by an anecdote: A woman in her thirties complained of both tennis elbow and carpal tunnel syndrome, both on her dominant side, persisting without remission over no less than 6 years. During this period she had had no relief from two steroid injections to each site or from surgical intervention, again to both sites. She had asymmetrical local physical signs in her neck, which had not been previously examined in 6 years, as well as tenderness at the elbow and the wrist, the latter presumably referred, in view of the fact that she was completely relieved of pain at both sites on a single manipulation of her neck! There was no history of abnormal electromyogram (EMG) or nerve conduction studies, nor did I instigate either of these. She was pain free.

Golfer's elbow is very similar to tennis elbow, in relation to the tendon insertions into the medial epicondyle of the humerus. The same considerations apply to both conditions in terms of diagnosis, the possibility of the pain being referred from the spine, potential problems, and management.

Carpal tunnel syndrome is usually ascribed to pressure on the median nerve in its passage through the carpal tunnel. It may present predominantly with pain, but paraesthesias in the hand and fingers are commonly reported. This condition often responds well to local anaesthetic and steroid injection, sometimes requiring surgery. However, like tennis elbow and golfer's elbow, it can also be referred from the lower cervical and upper thoracic spine. In the presence of abnormal local signs in the spine, it may well respond to suitable vertebral manipulation.

This is a strong argument in favour of local examination of the spine in all cases of pain in the arm, with vertebral manipulation as the first choice of therapy, in the absence of contraindication. In the event of no improvement resulting from taking this course, further tests, such as nerve conduction studies, are indicated. Usually of insidious inset, although sometimes related to trauma or known overuse, there is seldom anything surprising to be gained from the history in upper limb pain. The salient points are whether the patient feels ill, the precise site of pain, its mode of onset, whether it is intermittent or constant, whether it is accompanied by pain at other sites, and what activities or attempted activities make it worse or better.

As indicated above, local examination of the cervicothoracic spine should be regarded as mandatory in all cases of shoulder and arm pain. Its omission is a possible, if not probable, cause of failure of treatment.

Indications for cervicothoracic manipulation are the discovery of abnormal local physical signs, in the absence of contraindications.

Contraindications to cervicothoracic manipulation remain basically the same as described in Chapter 2. Strict adherence to them is fundamental to guaranteeing the exceptionally high level of safety of vertebral manipulation. In the absence of contraindication, discovery of asymmetry of local physical signs in the spine affords a presumptive diagnosis of simple spinal pain. If manipulation is chosen as the first treatment, the objective is twofold: the relief of pain and the concomitant remission of local physical signs. In view of the simplicity of the techniques involved, it would seem of advantage to the patient for the general practitioner to treat a substantial proportion of these problems on presentation.

Therapeutic techniques, even more than local examination techniques, demand the full educational process described in Chapter 6. It is no less than irresponsible to embark upon vertebral manipulation on the basis of reading alone.

Results are difficult to assess, but it is estimated that 30% of brachial pain is of spinal origin (15). This being the case, and in the light of the crude figures already reported, it is tempting to suggest that, in the presence of abnormal local physical signs and in the absence of contraindications to vertebral manipulation, a quick, noninvasive, safe therapy might be expected to produce encouraging results. In 40 years' experience, 15 of them in exclusively musculoskeletal practice, I can recollect but two instances in which I have worsened the patient's condition.

Chapter 10
Chest Pain

Anterior chest pain may arise from trauma that causes bruising or fracture of ribs. Diagnosis is commonly possible from the history, confirmed by palpation of the painful area, radiology seldom being required for clinical purposes, although perhaps indicated for medicolegal reasons. On the other hand, it may be the result of herpes zoster, pleurisy, Tietze's syndrome, coronary artery disease, pericarditis, or secondary carcinoma. In the first instance hyperaesthesia of the affected area is often sufficient to make the diagnosis prior to the appearance of the herpetic vesicles. Pleurisy may usually be diagnosed from the history and auscultation, again seldom requiring radiology for clinical purposes. It should be remembered that chest pain may be provoked by vigorous coughing, in the absence of pleurisy. Tietze's syndrome may be identified by clinical measures. Anterior chest pain is to be expected in coronary artery disease, with or without full-blown infarction, sometimes in association with neck or left arm pain. Pericarditis may be of insidious onset, not always easily identifiable clinically. Secondary carcinoma of a rib is again difficult to identify clinically, like the rare congenital cysts, often needing radiological confirmation. Asymmetry of local physical signs is unlikely in any of these conditions, in which there is no place for musculoskeletal procedures.

What is not widely known is that, in a series of several hundred cases of anterior chest pain simulating cardiac ischaemia, in which no changes were found on electrocardiogram (ECG), Fossgreen (16), a rheumatologist in Denmark, demonstrated abnormal local signs in the spine in a very substantial proportion of cases, most of them at or around the 4th thoracic segmental level. A high proportion of these patients were relieved of their pain by vertebral manipulation at the appropriate level. Cardiologists will agree that in about 20% of cases in which the pain suggests cardiac infarction, the ECG shows no abnormality. This is approximately the same incidence as

Fossgreen found in abnormal local physical signs. Is it the same 20%? This is not clear, but it is a very tempting proposition, which has not yet been shown to be wrong.

In addition to the causes cited for anterior chest pain, posterior thoracic pain may result from postural causes, particularly in those whose work demands stooping and lifting. While some of these cases will prove to be of simple muscular origin, in a proportion the pain will be accompanied by abnormal local signs, indicating local treatment. In addition to these cases, interscapular pain is a frequent accompaniment of cervical spinal abnormalities, as well as those of the thoracic spine. In the presence of local signs and in the absence of contraindications, encouraging results may be expected from cervical and/or thoracic vertebral manipulation. In the case of midthoracic girdle pain due to a centrally prolapsed intervertebral disc, all movements are likely to provoke pain – a clear contraindication to vertebral manipulation. Of course, women with excessively large breasts may experience thoracic pain. This is commonly relieved temporarily by lifting the breasts, and in the long term breast reduction may be considered.

Cervicothoracic spinal origins of thoracic pain are not at all uncommon, which lends weight to the advice that local examination of the whole spine should be regarded as mandatory, when any suspicion of a musculoskeletal problem exists. The fact that segmental nerve fibres may travel several segments up and down, both within the spinal cord and without, emphasizes the importance of this obligation.

History taking has been discussed already. It must be remembered that all patients edit their histories to some degree, many of them having preconceived ideas as to diagnosis, and it is essential for the doctor to ask relevant questions in order to elicit a fuller picture of the complaint. An anecdote illustrates this point: An elderly woman presented with unilateral chest pain of short duration, exacerbated by movement of the trunk. On direct questioning, she firmly denied any previous history of bony fracture, and her rib cage appeared reasonably mobile for a person of her age. But there were abnormal local signs on the right at the 6th thoracic level. In the absence of contraindications, I gently manipulated the appropriate level, whereupon she shrieked with pain, declaring that I had broken her rib, adding the gratuitous information that she had a congenital cyst in the rib in question and had suffered three previous fractures at the site over a number of years! Asked why she had not reported this fact on direct questioning, she replied that she did not think it mattered!

This emphasizes the importance of full history taking and meticulous data recording. As a result of her not being quite truthful when directly asked, there was, of course, no apparent indication for radiological investigation derived from her history and no contraindication to manipulation.

The local physical signs are the same as for the cervical spine, with the addition of the segmental sagittal pressure test and the lateral spinous process pressure test. These are illustrated in Chapter 2. It is worth reiterating that no one sign is diagnostic, but it is the sum of the abnormal local findings that indicates the site to which one should direct any local treatment, be it manipulation, local anaesthetic injection (with or without steroid), massage, transcutaneous electrical nerve stimulation (TENS), or acupuncture. Once again, accurate data recording is essential. An acceptable diagnostic term is suggested: pain of vertebral origin (PVO).

The examination of rib position and individual rib movements, which is widely taught, is of very dubious relevance, as is the attempted restoration of rib position or mobility by manipulation. There are three reasons for this statement. First, almost every rib has three articulations with four bony or cartilaginous structures, the rib head articulating with facets on two neighbouring vertebral bodies, the costovertebral articulation with the transverse process and the anterior articulation with the manubrium, the sternum, or via the costal cartilages. This makes detailed assessment more than complex. Second, pain from other sources, such as a posterior vertebral joint, almost invariably results in secondary alterations of rib-cage mobility between the two sides. Third, it is easy for the patient with good neuromuscular control to "cheat" by deliberately expanding one side of the chest more than the other! Of course, if vertebral manipulation resolves the patient's pain, more nearly symmetrical movement of the rib cage is likely to be restored. Nonetheless, it is still difficult to justify the claim that the cause of the pain was the observed asymmetry of movement.

Apart from the negative ECG findings discussed, other investigations may prove negative. For example, erythrocyte sedimention rate (ESR) may be normal in polymyalgia rheumatica, effectively denying the patient pertinent treatment (as I know to my cost!). And radiology may fail to reveal very early bony secondaries or the most minute of fractures.

Contraindications to thoracic vertebral manipulation are as for the rest of the spine, with the exception of the special considerations in the neck. There are no added contraindications for the thoracic region. The absolute contraindications are two. The first is rheumatoid arthritis. The reason for this is that while manipulation may give temporary relief, it inevitably delays the commencement of more appropriate treatment. The second is thoracic myelopathy, in which the vascular supply to the spinal cord is already poor, and may be worsened by even the most gentle, tentative manipulation.

The relative contraindications to vertebral manipulation are three. First, if all movements or attempted movements cause exacerbation of pain, then therapies other than manipulation should be employed. For the general practitioner, these include oral analgesics, gentle traction, local anaesthetic injection (with or without steroid), TENS, and acupuncture. Second, if the spine is grossly stiff, the same applies. Third, if, on "taking up the slack," the patient complains of appreciable pain, that particular manoeuvre should not be pursued. This latter is possibly the most useful contraindication, as vertebral manipulation should always be gentle, and the use of too great a force is unkind, unnecessary, and potentially dangerous (as mentioned earlier in the discussion of the employment of manipulation under general anaesthesia – it introduces a new, quite unnecessary risk).

Manipulative techniques are necessarily less precise in the thoracic spine than elsewhere, in view of the fact that the rib cage must have some splinting effect on all movements. The same restrictions on learning and practicing these techniques apply in this region as in the rest of the spine. The fantasy of specific manipulation is perhaps best illustrated in this region. It must be recognized as such and shunned.

Injection techniques present few problems; they are local anaesthetic and steroid injections to rib fractures, similar injections to trigger points (chiefly found at the medial margins of the scapulae), and the same to the posterior vertebral joints. It is not necessary to enter these joints, as emphasized earlier, but it is important to take the needle to the point of touching bone, so as to exclude the possibility of it being misplaced, possibly entering a blood vessel. Routine x-ray is not indicated, except in the case of doubt as to cause.

Results to be expected are good, though perhaps not so dramatically so as in the neck.

Chapter 11
Lower Trunk Pain

Posterior lower trunk pain is perhaps the commonest and best known of the whole body; it is lumbago. Although perhaps out-dated, *lumbago* is a term still used by many patients for the common, posterior examples of trunk pain. Of course, it is no more than a topographical label as to where the patient feels pain; it is neither a diagnosis nor a disease. Together with leg pain, it accounts for about 60% of pain of vertebral origin (PVO) and is of enormous importance as a cause of disability and loss of earnings (8). Even more than with posterior thoracic pain, low back pain is commonly related to stooping and lifting, to which may be added vibration. Not uncommonly it is accompanied or followed by pain in the sacroiliac region, the buttock, or the leg (the latter chiefly in the distribution of the greater sciatic nerve), in this circumstance almost always confined to one leg.

In spite of wide variations in history of onset, the site of origin of low back pain is usually found on local examination of the lumbar spine (although sometimes it is referred from the lower thoracic spine), in the form of asymmetry of the signs already described and illustrated. In the absence of contraindication, ver-tebral manipulation is the treatment of choice for simple low back pain, with injection in the vicinity of the posterior vertebral joints as the first choice of backup therapy. Other than those found along the iliac crests, trigger points are less common than they are higher up, requiring similar treatment.

However, it must be remembered that posterior trunk pain may be due to systemic causes, such as rheumatoid arthritis, in which case it should be remembered that this condition com-monly affects the sacroiliac joints early in its development. Pain may persist as low as this following polymyalgia rheumatica. It may also be referred from the kidney, when the pain is again likely to be unilateral. It is still frequently ascribed to interverte-bral disc protrusion, although this has been shown to be a rela-tively rare cause. It can be due to spinal stenosis. The possibility of myeloma cannot be ignored, nor that of Scheuermann's disease, in which Schmorl's nodes, while usually quite small and thus of little structural significance, may be large enough to seriously weaken the vertebral body. Vertebral manipulation is contraindicated in these conditions.

Though not so widely appreciated, anterior trunk pain is not uncommon, and it may lead to much diagnostic confusion. For example, epigastric pain can arise as high as the 6th thoracic level, apparent gallbladder pain at the seventh, renal pain at the eighth, and suprapubic pain as high as the tenth and eleventh. Pain in the inguinal fossa may be referred from the thoracolumbar segments, in addition to those derived from abdominal nerve entrapment syndrome, or nerve entrapment arising in herniorrhaphy scars. It is tempting to suggest that the occasional removal of a perfectly normal appendix may indeed be an illustration of this confusion. But to claim, as some complementary practitioners do, to treat acute appendicitis successfully by vertebral manipulation would be ludicrous, were it not dangerous. If right inguinal fossa pain is referred from the thoracolumbar spine, it is likely to be accompanied by abnormal local signs in the spine, in addition to the tenderness and muscle guarding to be expected at the site of perception of pain. Local physical signs need to be sought as a routine in these cases.

Similar claims are sometimes made in respect to other systemic diseases. These claims must be shunned. Nonetheless, it is surely a wise precaution to have the patient turn over, if in any doubt at all, and to look for local signs. Indeed it seems reasonable to look for abnormal local signs in the spine as a routine in patients presenting with abdominal pain; a number of unnecessary and ineffective surgical procedures may thus be avoided. Similarly, referred pain can cause confusion in other gut conditions, such as diverticulosis and irritable bowel syndrome, and possibly in gynaecological conditions. Although the causes of these pains are not within the province of musculoskeletal medicine, failure to examine the thoracolumbar spine locally may result in unnecessary suffering for the patient. In the absence of contraindications and in the presence of asymmetry of local signs, vertebral manipulation is worth consideration and quite likely to give early relief.

History taking is important in lower trunk pain, in particular in respect of possible concomitant mechanical and systemic causes for the symptoms. The patient with mechanically induced pain is unlikely to feel ill, while the patient with renal disease may well have a significant history. It is important to ask about digestive, urinary, and gynecological symptoms, as the patient may not volunteer them. In particular it is vital in these cases, as in those with leg or pelvic pain, to determine whether the patient has difficulty in micturition or saddle anaesthesia. Patients might not volunteer these symptoms, thinking them irrelevant, and might not report the latter on examination. These symptoms are in fact indications for immediate surgical referral, as they may indicate central compression of the spinal cord, which could result in lasting, major disability. Of course, sudden onset on a lifting strain makes a mechanical cause more likely, but it is unwise to rely on this.

The local signs to be sought are the same as previously described: skin pinching, assessment of muscle tone, search for trigger points, segmental sagittal pressure test, and lateral spinous process pressure test. Again, these demand patient cooperation, in that the patient is involved in reporting differences in discomfort on each test and at every level. It must be remembered that asymmetry of local signs should be sought anteriorly as well as posteriorly. Saddle anaesthesia must be sought a second time on examination and the patient again questioned about its presence. Data recording must be meticulous.

The contraindications to vertebral manipulation are the same as previously described, with the addition of the discovery of urinary problems and saddle anaesthesia, the latter demanding urgent surgical referral.

Results of lumbar manipulation are commonly fairly encouraging. In the trial of 1037 patients previously quoted, 36.3% of the lumbar group of 673 patients were pain free in one session, a further 21.9% in a second, and 8.1% more in a third session (8).

Traction may be of use, in which case it may be worthwhile using a modified version of the apparatus described in Chapter 8. As will be seen from the illustration, the spreader bar is the same as that for cervical traction, but now is used in conjunction with two swivel bars, so as to permit the sharing of weight between the head and the axillae. The head harness is the same, but two axillary loops are added, each adjustable, in order to take into account the differences in distance of level of the chin and the axillae to be found between patients. This adjustment requires the assistance of the physician, but subsequently patients may apply traction as and when they find it suitable.

As in cervical traction, the height at which the apparatus is hung should permit the head harness to be put on while the patient is standing comfortably. The patient should then put his

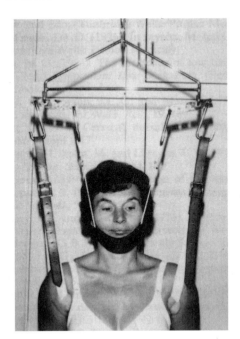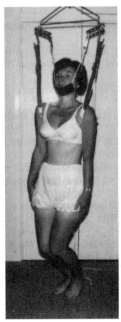

FIGURE 11.1. DIY lumbar traction apparatus. (From Paterson JK, Burn L. *An Introduction to Medical Manipulation*. Lancaster, England: MTP Press, 1985, p. 181.)

arms through the axillary loops, (padding them suitably for comfort). Provided that the axillary loops have been correctly adjusted, the swivel bars of the apparatus should be roughly horizontal. These bars have five holes for spreader and hooks at one-inch centres. If the apparatus is assembled as shown, it will be apparent that three eighths of any pull applied will be taken on each axilla, and one quarter on the neck. Traction may be applied by patient sagging at the knee, going so far as to take his feet off the ground, if he feels so inclined. Again, he can apply traction for as long a period as he may choose, and repeat it several times at a session – always remembering to ease the strain gently. With the apparatus in the home, it is possible to apply traction several times a day, and the countereffects of driving home after treatment are avoided (Figs. 11.1 and 11.2).

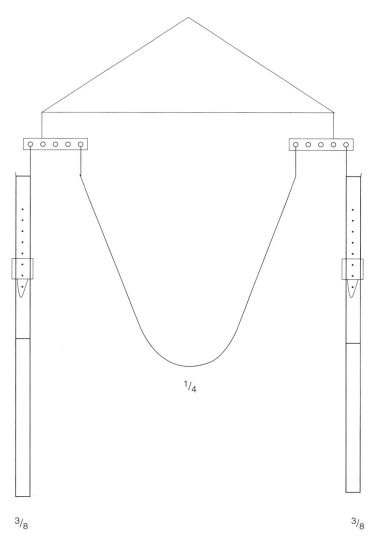

FIGURE 11.2. DIY lumbar traction diagram.

Chapter 12
Pelvic Pain

The significance and diagnostic pitfalls of inguinal fossa pain has been discussed in the previous chapter, in which epigastric, gall-bladder, renal, ureteric, and bladder pain have also been mentioned. Each has its particular history and attendant physical signs, but the common reality of referred pain does not exclude the possibility of pains at any of these sites being of mechanical origin, most likely arising between the 8th and 12th thoracic levels, as well as the lumbar ones, even when systemic disease is at first suspected. It is equally important to remember that the teaching of cure of any of these conditions by manipulation remains a dangerous dream. So to the pelvis itself.

As previously mentioned, the pubic bones, like every other structure in the skeleton, may not be symmetrical in form; indeed they are seldom so. This may result in their appearing not to be level on the two sides. Therefore, clinically observed differences in level must be of no diagnostic value. Such an observation does not imply any degree of malposition. Of course, this does not mean that it is useless to observe the apparent differences, before and after manipulation. It must be remembered that the symphysis has a disc somewhat similar to the intervertebral disc, and that it may be damaged by excessive stresses. Other than in complex traffic accidents, where in any case manipulative techniques would not be contemplated, such damage is rare, though less so during and following pregnancy, as a result of the physiological slackening of all the pelvic ligaments. In the latter case it is associated with the distraction force of the infant's head, due to uterine muscular contraction during the second stage of labour in effect prizing open the pelvic outlet. Other than these cases, I have seen one case in 40 years of musculoskeletal practice; it was due to trauma by the pommel of a saddle, in a horseman misjudging a jump. A sudden upward blow to the converging inferior pubic rami put a distraction force on the symphysis sufficient to separate it by disruption of the disc. It is noteworthy that the causative force in this case is diametrically opposed to that in intervertebral disc rupture – distraction, rather than compression.

One of the commonest pelvic pains is that felt over the sacroiliac joints. The possibility of this being due to rheumatoid arthritis or Scheuermann's disease has already been mentioned, as has polymyalgia rheumatica. While the same principles apply here in pregnancy as at the symphysis pubis, the suggestion that the sacroiliac joints are common sites of origin of (nonpregnancy) musculoskeletal problems requires further thought. There are three cogent reasons for viewing this unsubstantiated belief with grave suspicion. First, the sacroiliac joints are the largest joints in the body, irregular in shape, and their articular surfaces are deeply pitted, with compensatory prominences engaging in the pits, so that their interlocking allows minimal movement, except under a strong distraction force between the ileum and sacrum. Application of such a force just does not occur, except in the second stage of labour or complex accidental trauma.

Second, they are supported by the largest and strongest ligaments in the entire body, keeping the deep pits and prominences very firmly engaged, by this means restricting movement even more.

Third, they have been shown to be a common site for referred pain from the lumbar spine, or from the thoracolumbar junction, though most often from the fourth and fifth lumbar and the first sacral posterior joints.

Thus the widely canvassed notional diagnosis of the sacroiliac lesion seems to be at best dubious – indeed little more than a fantasy! It is certainly not proven. Further, there are several therapeutic techniques taught to correct the assumed restriction or displacement of these joints – mainly osteopathic or chiropractic. It is highly significant that, in the employment of every one of these techniques, a great many other structures are stressed and/or moved, including the posterior spinal joints known to commonly give rise to referred pain at these sites. In view of their structure, the sacroiliac joints must be the least likely of the entire skeletal system to suffer displacement and the least likely to be moved therapeutically, and their most important feature is that their movement is very restricted for a start!

History taking has already been discussed in relation to the numerous systemic diseases likely to cause confusion. By far the most important two items in assessment must be saddle anaesthesia and disturbances of micturition. These are, of course, absolute contraindications to mechanical intervention, demanding immediate surgical referral. It also remains important to keep in mind both the manner of history taking – asking the right questions in words the patient can understand – and its recording (see Chapter 2).

Unlike the sacroiliac joints, the coccyx is not uncommonly displaced, being attached to the skeleton at one extreme, rather than being sandwiched between two other bony structures. It also has relatively weak supporting ligaments, and from time to time is subjected to trauma of one sort or another, including the second stage of labour. Although widely regarded as being difficult to treat (most often this is by injection, though quite commonly with disappointing results), coccydynia is sometimes rapidly relieved by manipulation – a procedure not entirely pleasant for either the patient or the physician, but often effective! This is the only painful manipulative technique that should be tolerated, as the increased pain is of very brief duration, no damage can result from it, and relief is usually immediate, which makes the procedure worthwhile in spite of the transient pain it may cause. It is important to tell the patient to expect a sharp pain.

Local physical signs are again as previously described, in addition to those of routine orthopaedic and neurological origin. They are skin pinching, assessment of paravertebral muscle tone, a search for trigger points, segmental sagittal pressure, lateral spinous process pressure, a search for zygoapophyseal tenderness, iliac separation, iliac crest compression, and sacral thrust. These are illustrated in Chapter 2.

Contraindications are as already described.

Therapeutic techniques remain essentially simple and far from specific. In view of what has been said above, manipulative techniques are only indicated where there are no contraindications, and when pelvic pain is accompanied by local spinal signs – generally they are low thoracic and lumbar techniques, with the one possible addition mentioned above, that of manipulation of the coccyx.

Results from manipulation, including those for the trunk, pelvis, and leg, are fairly encouraging, although not so good as for the cervical region. In the trial of 1037 patients previously quoted, 36.3% of the 673-patient lumbar group were pain free in on session, a further 21.9% in a second, and 8.1% more in a third.

Chapter 13
Leg Pain

Together with lumbar pain, leg pain accounts for about two thirds of all pain of vertebral origin (PVO). Ignoring pain arising in the hip, knee, ankle, and foot, a substantial proportion of leg pain is found in the distribution of the greater sciatic nerve. Astonishingly, it is still widely believed that disc protrusion is responsible for the majority of cases of lumbar and leg pain. One source put the figure at 95% (23). Yet it has been shown that appreciable disc protrusions are to be found in no less than 37% of patients who do not currently have and never have had back or leg pain (53). And, in no way reflecting upon the skill of the surgeon, it is not an uncommon finding for no clinical benefit to follow surgical "cure" of a demonstrable protrusion (54). The inference that has to be drawn from these facts is clear: such a belief is unsound.

Although sciatic pain is a common accompaniment of lumbar pain, either can exist on its own. Anterior leg pain is relatively uncommon, again with no clear correlation between it and lumbar pain. However, it is important to remember that gluteal and leg pain can arise higher in the spinal column than might be expected, not infrequently at the thoracolumbar junction, and indeed, quite aside from the phenomenon of referred pain, the posterior rami of L1 an L2 have been shown to cross the pelvic brim, penetrating well into the buttock (14). Too great a reliance on charts of segmental innervation is inadvisable (see Chapter 2).

A further point of importance lies in the changes in shape, positioning, and movement of the intervertebral disc that occur on changes of pressure applied to it – some physiological, others pathological. Obviously, in view of the fact that the nucleus pulposus, being semifluid, is incompressible, any variation in applied pressure must distort the annulus fibrosus. Such distortion may be bilaterally symmetrical, in which case the disc is acting simply as a shock absorber. Or it may be asymmetrical, dependent on any coexistent flexion, extension, side bending, or rotation. In either case, the distortion is directly related in degree to the pressure applied. Of course, to some extent this is normal, so as to permit intervertebral movement, but when the annular and ligamentous distortion is excessive, perhaps due to local variations in their weakening, pressure on a nerve root or on the spinal cord may ensue. A weakened annulus fibrosus, together with a weakening of its supporting ligaments, will bulge the more on an increase of pressure put on any mobile spinal segment. Of course, marked weakening of both structures is the precursor of rupture of the annulus fibrosus. Therefore, any activity that increases intradiscal pressure is potentially harmful, and maybe seriously so. Some may be surprised to learn that the activity that causes the greatest increase in intradiscal pressure is the sit-up, one of the commonest exercises prescribed today (38). Fitness fanatics and their clubs and institutes take note! The evidence has been available for a quarter of a century.

The history is variable. As already described, some lumbar pain is of dramatically sudden onset, commonly on excessively vigorous movement under load, while in other cases it is insidious, apparently lacking correlation with any known factor. Sudden onset of leg pain is less common. It has been widely taught that the sudden-onset cases respond better to manipulative techniques than do the insidious onset ones. In view of the findings in the unselected series quoted, it seems unlikely that this is the case (8). Like lumbar pain, leg pain is commonly recurrent. However, the belief that it is likely to get progressively worse or more frequent with advancing years is just not true; the incidence actually declines significantly after the age of 55 (55).

As in all regions, local examination is necessary in addition to standard orthopaedic and neurological examination. The basic techniques are as detailed in Chapter 2. It is emphasized that standardized data recording saves time for the physician and greatly improves the quality of material available for research purposes.

It is worth noting that too great a reliance on differences in straight leg raising can be misleading, such differences being common in asymptomatic patients as well as in those with posterior compartment syndrome. It is further important to note that appreciable differences in leg length are commonly normal for the individual. This raises another question: How is leg length best measured? Several methods are currently in use. First, the tape-measure distance from the anterior superior iliac spine to the medial malleolus of the tibia is not a measure of leg length at all, as the distance measured is derived from both the length of the legs and the (probably asymmetrical) shape of the pelvis; the distance measured gives a false impression of equality or inequality of leg length. Second, radiological measurement of leg length differences is accurate, but pelvic asymmetry is just as likely to cause effective differences in relation to posture. While revealing the true leg length difference, it does not assess the effective difference. Its relevance is therefore dubious. Third, the common use of "sighting," with the examiner's forefingers laid along the iliac crests, checking against an observed horizontal line, is no better.

There is a fourth method, which provides an accurate measure of the effective difference in leg length in relation to the spine. Estimation of the lateral index of sacral tilt (LIST) is based on the reasonable proposition that any angle from the horizontal that the upper surface of the sacrum assumes in the antero-posterior view is likely to adversely influence the incidence of PVO, through the asymmetry of mechanical stresses imposed by the compensatory scoliosis induced (42). As this angle is likely to be quite small, its precise measurement is a problem. More accurate and clinically useful results are obtained by using the trigonometric tangent of that angle, with the added advantage that one of the measurements made is the effective difference in leg length. The method is described in detail in the references cited, and a brief account follows.

An x-ray of the lumbar spine is taken in the anteroposterior view, with the patient standing, his toes turned in to encourage equal weight bearing on the two sides. Horizontal lines are drawn on the x-ray through the highest points of each femoral head. Vertical lines are drawn through the points of contact of each horizontal line with the femoral heads. The vertical distance between these two horizontal lines is the true leg length difference (Fig. 13.1).

Next, a line is drawn through the lumbosacral joint, intersecting with both vertical lines, thus revealing any slope there may be to the platform on which the lumbar spine is based. A third horizontal line is drawn through the intersection of the sloping line with one of the vertical lines. The angle between these lines is the angle of slope from the horizontal, but this may be difficult to measure accurately. What is easy to measure is the vertical distance between the third horizontal line and the sloping line, x, and the distance between the two vertical lines, y, the former being the effective difference in leg length (Fig. 13.2).

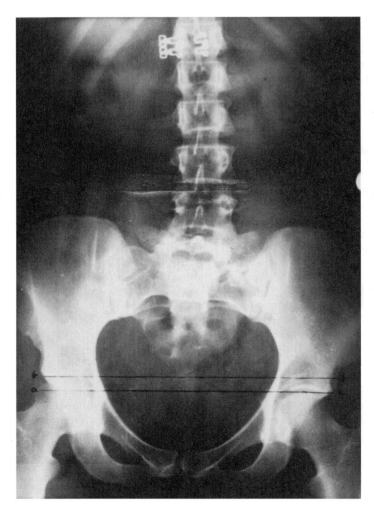

FIGURE 13.1. True leg length difference – radiological.

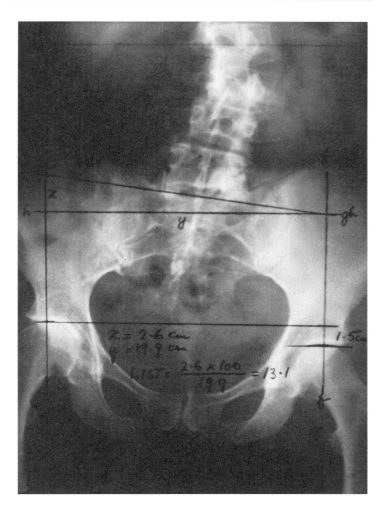

FIGURE 13.2. Lateral index of sacral tilt – radiograph.

The LIST is recorded as x multiplied by 100, divided by y. A markedly asymmetrical example is shown (Figs. 13.3 and 13.4).

It is interesting that, while leg length differences may be the root of spinal problems, in numerous instances no disability is suffered, and substantial differences may result in minimal disability. One Olympic speed skater had an effective difference of

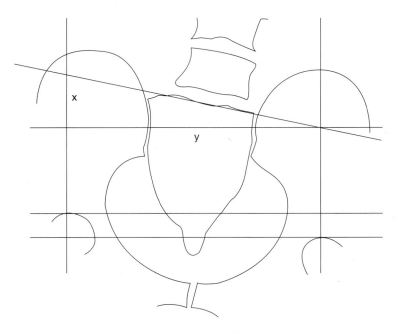

FIGURE 13.3. Lateral index of sacral tilt – diagram.

5.5 cm (happily shorter on the inside of the bends), while a marathon runner of the "third age,"[1] at the time ranked fifth in the world, had a difference of 6.5 cm, of which he was wholly unaware! Neither of these patients required treatment. When it comes to clinical management, as most patients will have accommodated for this difference over a period of several years, it is probably best to commence treatment with a heel raise of half the height demonstrated by LIST. If the raise is considerable, the sole must also be raised to some degree.

Contraindications for manipulation in cases of leg pain are as for the rest of the spine, with the particular addition of saddle anaesthesia and disturbance of micturition.

Once again, therapeutic techniques must be learned properly. Most of the manipulative techniques are similar in principle to those employed higher up the spine, but it is reiterated that learning solely from a book is a recipe for disaster. In all these techniques it is the taking up of the slack prior to any thrust that is the ultimate key to safe and effective practice.

[1] The above mentional "third age" refers to people over the age of 65 years.

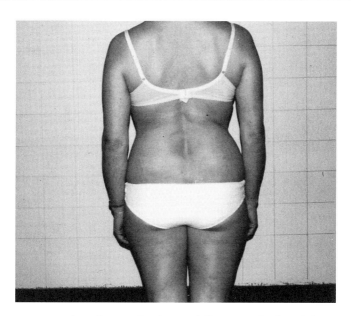

FIGURE 13.4. Clinical example of gross difference in leg length.[2]

Traction may be valuable. In this case it is worth considering the apparatus described in Chapter 11. It is stressed that domiciliary use avoids the necessity for patients to travel to and from the physician's office or the hospital, often in considerable discomfort, not infrequently undoing any good their treatment may have done.

The injections applicable to leg pain are to trigger points and to the posterior vertebral joints, to which may be added caudal epidurals. The reasons for restricting the latter to the caudal route are two. First, they are easier to perform than their lumbar counterparts, and second, they are much safer, so long as they are done with care. They are thus better suited to use in general practice. As already noted, it is vital that these injections should

[2] Observations regarding Figure 13.4: The indentation of outline at waist level is less pronounced on the left than on the right. The point of maximum indentation is lower on the left than on the right. The lumbar spine is killed to the left. The lower thoracic spine reveals a compensatory bend to the right. The left shoulder is lower than the right shoulder. The patient has a short left leg.

be undertaken only when adequate resuscitation facilities are immediately to hand. They are easy to learn, as are their attendant potential problems, but again they should not be attempted without proper instruction. In several thousand such injections, I have failed to penetrate the sacral hiatus on one occasion and had great difficulty on one other, the latter due to the substantial obesity of the patient; finding the sacral cornua at all was extremely difficult! I have had one case in which there was brief hypotension, in a patient who had failed to answer truthfully to my routine question as to a history of local anaesthetic mishap; he had had previous trouble with dental anaesthesia. Happily, this solitary case responded well to the immediate administration of adrenaline.

There remain some who use up to 50 mL in epidural injections. Not only is this unnecessary, as, contrary to some quite forceful teaching, local anaesthetic and steroid molecules pass rapidly through the dura into the epidural fluid, reaching the brain rapidly, but it is unkind and wasteful; 10 mL is frequently enough, and a few cases warrant 20 mL.

One cause of failure with caudal epidurals is the presence of scar tissue in the spinal canal, especially after surgery. In view of the technical difficulties involved in lumbar epidural injections, I would discourage the family doctor from employing the latter techniques. Likewise, procedures like epidurography and epiduroscopy are matters for referral.

Results to be expected are as reported in Chapter 12.

Chapter 14
Will Musculoskeletal Medicine Work?

Vertebral manipulation lies at the heart of musculoskeletal medicine. Indeed, I wonder why the term *manual medicine* has been so widely dropped? Perhaps some felt it was in some way degrading for a professional – rather akin to manual labour. At least it suggested the most likely approach to the patient's problem – primarily by the use of the hands. Either way, many musculoskeletal patients expect manipulation as a first choice of therapy, and, not unreasonably, they want to know whether it is going to work. This expectation is enhanced by today's trend toward evidence-based medicine.

As previously indicated, manipulation is not for every patient. What chiefly distinguishes bone setters from musculoskeletal practitioners is that the latter, if properly taught, are acutely aware of what they must avoid, whereas the former can but operate on a rather hit-and-miss basis. Even in the 21st century, there are numerous alternative practitioners to be found, some calling themselves osteopaths, some chiropractors of one sort or another (some without the support of a proper qualification), while there remain in rural areas a number of old-fashioned bone setters. It is interesting that, certainly widely in India, cervical manipulation is commonly carried out by barbers – as an optional extra to a haircut. And jolly refreshing it is, too! Those who have experienced this will recollect that their postmanipulative posture is dramatically altered – they stand tall!

As already described, the contraindications to vertebral manipulation are absolute and relative in every spinal region, and the manipulator's comprehensive knowledge and rigid observation of them is vital to the safety of the patient. It is not so much a matter of which techniques to avoid as which patients need to be protected from mechanical procedures entirely. In fact it is difficult to imagine an intrinsically dangerous manipulation, except under general anaesthesia (see Chapter 6). Rather, the dangers lie in manipulating the wrong patient. But the patient will still quite reasonably want to know whether the intended therapy will work.

Injections have been described previously, largely as a second string to the manipulator's bow. These may be the first choice, as in the presence of contraindications to manipulation, as much as the second choice on manipulation not producing the desired result in a very short time. In either case patients may well ask whether the injection is going to work. After all, it is their pain that is under consideration! And of course, as mentioned previously, unlike the situation with the bone setter, there are other treatments available to the musculoskeletal practitioner. The point has already been made that adequate resuscitation facilities must be immediately available, particularly when employing caudal epidural anaesthesia, which may be called upon in emergency. Also, the practitioner must have in readiness adrenaline, a spare syringe, and swabs for immediate use – not just their availability somewhere in the building. I would strongly advise against any route other than the caudal in general practice.

Of course, it is perfectly reasonable for the patient to wish to know whether any proposed musculoskeletal treatment is going to work. In spite of widespread teaching to the contrary, the hard truth is that this is seldom possible to foretell with any certainty. Every musculoskeletal technique is indeed to some extent empirical (55). This news is not very well received by some – patients and doctors alike. But I have found few patients who will not accept this fundamental truth, so long as it is presented in a sober, down-to-earth manner, backed by two assurances. First, patients need to know that what is proposed can do them no harm. With an adequate history and the rigid observance of the contraindications, this is almost invariably predictable. Second, they need to know that there are alternative therapies available, should the one first proposed fail to help. Most distressed by this truth are those who make a habit of making such predictions! They include a number of orthodox medical practitioners, as well as declared complementary ones. All such unsubstantiated therapeutic predictions as to outcome need to be taken with a large pinch of salt! They are more than likely to be proved wrong. And they are potentially dangerous on a second count, as they may delay the prescription of a more appropriate treatment.

Perhaps worse than rash predictions as to efficacy of any particular therapy is the unwarranted prescription of a specified number of treatments sometimes met with - in some quarters, mostly amongst chiropractors, it is not uncommon for a patient on first attendance to be recommended a course of a dozen treatments. In view of the crude figures quoted earlier in this book, showing a high proportion of patients relieved of their symptoms in a single treatment, with substantially more in three treatments (8), this is clearly not in the interests of the patient, though it may help swell the income of the practitioner concerned.

This brings us to the question of cost, which is of interest to the patient, the general practitioner, the hospital physician, the various medical provident associations, and the taxpayer. The answer is self-evident. If musculoskeletal therapies are unpredictable in outcome, there can be no justification in adding to the cost by prescribing a long series of treatments; rather, practitioners must be prepared to change their tactics after no more than three attempts, in the event that their first therapeutic choice proves of little or no help at this stage. Few are the patients who will not accept the wisdom and honesty of this approach and its economic desirability.

Immediate posttherapeutic assessment of the patient is mandatory after every procedure, in order to compare the situation with that prior to treatment. In the case of vertebral manipulation, alteration in signs may be immediate, as may be alteration in symptoms, but patients must be told that there can be no guarantee that this will prove the case in the longer term. They must be impressed that follow-up is essential, even if only one visit![1]

One eminent teacher of osteopathy frequently declared, "I can tell," in a variety of contexts. One musculoskeletal physician of international stature assured countless patients, "We'll soon put you right." What is clear is that these two declarations, one of diagnostic ability, the other of predicted outcome, are unscientific, misleading and potentially to the detriment of the patient. Little seems to have changed. A measure of honesty is indicated.

[1]Again, in the UK this implies a domiciliary visit.

Chapter 15
The Future of Musculoskeletal Medicine

Musculoskeletal medicine has previously been defined, and its admittedly limited scientific bases have been spelled out. It has been viewed through the eyes of the patient and of the physician, and the important aspect of its economics has been addressed. Its teaching within the orthodox fold has been discussed, with particular emphasis on how easily and quickly this may be achieved, provided techniques are simplified and limited in number, and that all tenets of faith are eschewed, in favour of such valid evidence as has been adduced. Distribution of pain commonly associated with it has been discussed, in particular the phenomenon of referred pain, together with its twin, referred tenderness. Consideration has been given to the vexing question as to whether or not vertebral manipulation, its therapeutic core, will work for the individual patient. No practitioner should contemplate such a prediction! Nor should any patient accept such advice. Apart from the shoulder, elbow, carpal tunnel, and leg, the application of manipulation to peripheral structures has been deliberately omitted, as these aspects of musculoskeletal medicine are perhaps even less acceptable to orthodox practitioners.

It is important to look squarely to the future. But to obtain a balanced view, it is advisable first to recapitulate something of musculoskeletal medicine's history. In the first place, quite apart from its employment in ancient Egypt, the Far East, and elsewhere over thousands of years, vertebral manipulation, the basic therapy in this field, was taught and practiced by Hippocrates, rendering it orthodox from the very beginnings of Western medicine. Thus, justification for regarding it as necessarily alternative or complementary is frankly scant. For some unknown reason it was lost to the medical profession for a very long time, in the United Kingdom becoming, by orthodox default, the domain of the bone setters.

In 1874 it resurfaced in the United States with an ideology specifically alternative to orthodoxy; this was osteopathy. In sorrow and frustration over illness and deaths in his own family, which he felt should have been avoidable, Andrew Taylor Still, himself a doctor, became convinced that orthodox medicine was both wrong in its teaching and potentially harmful in its practice. Believing that God could never have intended the suffering he and his family experienced, he turned to religion. He evolved his own theories as to causation and cure of a number of illnesses, the core of his therapy being the restoration of normal (mainly spinal) joint mobility, which would cure all manner of diseases. This he taught with zeal. And these ideas he set out some years later in his autobiography (32). But, quite apart from not demonstrating any relationship between spinal joints and a variety of illnesses, he never demonstrated how modestly abnormal movement could be clinically discerned when, in the asymptomatic subject, range of movement varies as widely as it has since been shown to do. This remains a matter of faith. If you cannot identify normal range of movement, how can you substantiate an instance of the abnormal?

In 1895 a further alternative was offered, again in the U.S., this time by Daniel David Palmer, a schoolmaster turned grocer, believed to possess the power of healing. This was chiropractic, firmly based on Palmer's more extreme premise that all illness was derived from spinal malposition rather than asymmetry of movement, and was therefore best treated by vertebral manipulation, by putting the misplaced bones back in their proper places (29). In view of the related facts that no vertebra is perfectly symmetrical in form, and that no two vertebrae are identical in contour, it is difficult to see how anyone can clinically identify either normal alignment or malposition of individual vertebrae. What is easy to discern is differences in bony knobbiness at paired sites, which may be either normal or abnormal for the individual. How wrong Palmer is seen to have been!

These two ideologies are alternative in thought, word, and deed. They also embrace a welter of diagnostic and therapeutic techniques of daunting number and complexity, some of which have been discussed earlier in this book.

In 1932, on the evidence of but one case (22), Western medicine latched onto the concept that the cause of much of the pain presenting as a constituent part of musculoskeletal medicine lay in protrusion of the intervertebral disc, with consequent nerve root or spinal cord compression (23). Somehow this became widely referred to as the "slipped disc," a misleading idea, long since disproved, though still commonly promoted. In due course, such rather minor medical interest as there was in the broader field of musculoskeletal medicine became international, coming under the umbrella of the Fédération Internationale de Médecine Manuelle (FIMM). The British Association of Manual Medicine (BAMM) was set up in 1963, and over a number of years similar associations appeared in about 25 nations. Each association evolved its own particular philosophy, sometimes varying one from another surprisingly widely, though all substantially inclined in the direction of osteopathy or chiropractic, in preference to current orthodox teaching or nonteaching (1).

In 1986 the British Medical Association (BMA) published a review of alternative therapy (56). It is perhaps pertinent that the distinguished membership of the working party producing this short book did not, I believe, include a member with specific training or experience in vertebral manipulation, the most widely used therapy in this field. In its report the association referred to the medical manipulator as "an expensively trained specialist." As made clear already, the requisite training is not relatively expensive, a period of a solid year or more being quite unnecessary, and there remains serious doubt as to whether musculoskeletal medicine should be regarded as a specialty, as will be discussed shortly. The association also made this further statement: "Provided a medical diagnosis is first made, and the known contraindications to certain manipulations are respected, the registered lay manipulator probably provides the community with a generally safe and helpful service."

The BMA included in its brief bibliography of the field the first of the five texts written by Burn and myself (57), in which we set out the very limited, though clinically adequate, scientific bases of vertebral manipulation. As previously stated and wholly contrary to their second comment quoted above, a clinically provable diagnosis is seldom possible in musculoskeletal practice. The reasons for this are the complexities of the neuromuscular system, which permit identical pain to be felt emanating from a variety of anatomical sources, often far from the site of perception of pain, coupled with the phenomenon of muscle substitution, which commonly prevents accurate clinical identification of muscles at fault. More important, an assumed diagnosis can prove disastrous, as it may well lead to perpetuation of an inappropriate therapy, possibly wasting crucial time before the patient is more effectively treated.

On the other hand, a presumptive diagnosis is perfectly acceptable, provided one is prepared to change one's mind on the production of valid evidence showing the diagnosis to be unsound. And such a presumptive diagnosis may be derived from painstaking history taking and local examination, coupled with meticulous data recording. Further, there is currently no guarantee that the lay manipulator will know the contraindications – let alone respect them. The BMA report made no suggestion as to how such knowledge and respect might be assured.

In 1989, toward the end of my three-year presidency of BAMM, following eight years as honorary secretary, the FIMM triennial congress was held in London. This was complemented by a review text derived from 55 of the papers presented at the congress (1). Its first part opened with the presentation of the appropriate, proven scientific bases of musculoskeletal medicine by hard-line, nonmanipulating medical specialists: B. Lynn, G.B.J. Anderson, J.V. Basmajian, A.E. Reading, S. McMahon, and M.A. Nelson. It continued with 13 plenary papers from senior figures already in the musculoskeletal field, followed by 10 directed papers and 26 free papers. This pattern highlighted the wide differences in teaching existing between member countries of FIMM, also revealing a sorry lack of general adherence to proven fact. This review was closely followed by a further and much fuller, copiously referenced, science-based text (6). Not long after this congress, BAMM ceased to exist as a separate entity, becoming amalgamated with the British Institute of Musculoskeletal Medicine (BIMM).

In 1994 the Clinical Standards Advisory Committee published its very important, if somewhat superficial report on back pain (31). Perhaps the greatest importance of this report lay in its spelling out the dangers of manipulating the wrong spine, putting the contraindications in their rightfully prime place. It also made use of the term *simple back pain*. This document was strongly reinforced by a paper from the Royal College of General Practitioners (58). The latter report recognized that the preferred home of musculoskeletal medicine was in general practice. In 1995, as chairman of the Scientific Advisory Committee of FIMM, I published a further text, expressly as a working guide to a series of three international teachers' workshops I had been deputed to present (45). My remit was to coordinate musculoskeletal teaching internationally – on a sound scientific basis. In spite of many very welcome individual changes in attitude to differing aspects of the subject amongst those attending the workshops, I failed to consolidate these changes in the time available, due in good measure to determined opposition from some of those established as musculoskeletal "gurus," including the president of FIMM at the time! I suppose I was rocking the boat too much. Perhaps encouraged in part by the BMA report (56), for some years past BIMM has vigorously pursued a course aimed at achieving recognition of musculoskeletal medicine as a specialty. It continues this course to this day. To varying extents similar moves have been made in a number of member associations within FIMM, particularly in Germany and the United States. As yet, the international medical establishment has not welcomed this approach with any great enthusiasm. It is pertinent to ask why this has been the case. What have been their objections? Are these objections valid today?

There are four major objections to such a proposal. First, the great majority of medical practitioners employing vertebral manipulation, though necessarily qualified at a basic level, have not attained a higher qualification, such as membership of the Royal College of Physicians, surely a prerequisite to specialist status. Second, apart from those electing to seek overtly alternative help on their own initiative, the great majority of patients with musculoskeletal problems present in primary care, only a tiny proportion needing to proceed to hospital, mainly to departments of orthopaedic surgery or rheumatology, or, particularly in the case of patients with chronic pain, to pain clinics – and this usually after a considerable wait. Third, as has been stressed in Chapter 6, there is nothing difficult in learning the appropriate diagnostic, manipulative, and injection techniques, and their employment is safe, so long as the contraindications are constantly borne in mind and rigidly observed. The dangers must be fully appreciated, and the problem patients recognized and either treated in another manner or referred elsewhere. Fourth, no clear scientific advance in clinical diagnosis or treatment has been demonstrated; diagnostic techniques of necessity remain substantially subjective, while therapeutic techniques are thousands of years old.

Assuming these four objections to be valid – and I have yet to hear any sound evidence to the contrary – the size of the problem, in excess of 20% of the general practitioner's work load, surely calls for the inclusion of the basic elements of musculoskeletal medicine in the undergraduate curriculum, and the postgraduate curriculum needs to offer further pursuit of this domain to those who wish to enjoy it (3). The fact that about 50% of undergraduate medical students are probably destined for primary care lends emphasis to this proposition. But, of course, this necessitates a small addition to the undergraduate course load.

There will be many medical educators horrified at the prospect of yet another subject being crammed into an already overloaded curriculum, but the extent of the problem and the ease with which this clearly demonstrated educational void may be filled surely demand further consideration of this stance. Too many patients are suffering unnecessarily, for want of sober understanding of the field by the medical profession – in the first place by general practitioners, but also by all those members of recognised specialist departments who may encounter the primary care failures at a later stage. It follows that the same considerations apply to postgraduate as to undergraduate teaching.

A further matter is worthy of consideration at this point. Both FIMM and BIMM have recently altered their statutes so as to admit to membership applicants without medical qualification. In so doing they have rendered themselves no longer exclusively representative of the medical profession. How this may be aligned with claims to medical specialty status of musculoskeletal medicine is difficult to grasp. But it does not detract from the importance of the field from the patient's point of view.

Given that the dangers are appreciated from the outset, and that the contraindications are observed rigidly, the advantages to the patient of being treated in primary care are two. First, he is likely to be relieved of his symptoms much earlier than he would otherwise be. Second, the overall therapeutic cost is likely to be dramatically reduced. Surely, the best deal for the patient on both these scores has to be the relatively inexpensive learning of the basic skills by at least one member of the primary care team, not excluding physiotherapists, enabling the practice to cope effectively with the substantial majority of these cases on the spot, without recourse to hospitals or complementary personnel. This is wholly contrary to the view expressed in the BMA publication quoted, but over at least 15 years it has been found to work well in the relatively few instances of such a policy having been adopted. One manual (5), previously thoroughly read, with the addition of three $1^1/_2$-day practical postgraduate courses, largely for GPs, is likely to benefit the patient, the taxpayer, the provident associations, and the primary care team, and to relieve the hospitals of a substantial clinical burden they are often today ill-fitted to shoulder. And they have better things to do with their time!

It follows that, in addition to the desirability of the entire medical profession having a broad understanding of musculoskeletal medicine, all specialist departments to which the relatively few primary care failures might be referred should be prepared and equipped to make use of its techniques when the occasion arises, as there will inevitably be some cases of simple back pain that slip through the net of primary care. This could most readily be achieved by the medical profession discarding once and for all the tenets of alternativism and taking over musculoskeletal medicine as an integral part of the establishment.

In practice this first entails teaching undergraduates the simple bases of the epidemiology of pain of vertebral origin, pain perception and modulation (including mention of the psychological aspects of pain), the relevant anatomy, the relevant pathology, and the indications and contraindications for vertebral manipulation. This needs to be complemented by a sound grounding in history taking and local examination. Second, it involves making brief practical courses more widely available to postgraduates, coupled with suitable financial inducements. With the active cooperation of the Royal Colleges, particularly that of the Royal College of General Practitioners, in conjunction with the deans of medical schools, this should prove a simple and effective means of putting an end to a long-standing and expensive argument within the profession. It is heartening to know that the Royal College of General Practitioners has already identified this field as demanding early appraisal (59).

In view of the evidence currently available, seen to be strongly in favour of reintegration of basic musculoskeletal medicine into the orthodox primary care fold, there seems but slender call for yet another specialty. What is required is surely a special interest group within primary care.

Envoi

Although this short book is written primarily in respect to practice within the United Kingdom, it is worth noting that other countries, and even the Council of Europe, are concerned about the current, ongoing situation regarding musculoskeletal medicine. In a recent short resolution by the Parliamentary Assembly, comments and recommendation were made that demand close examination. While this resolution was made in respect to a wider range of nonconventional medicine, it made particular reference to osteopathy and chiropractic (60).

It was noted that "alternative, complementary and other forms of medicine" were "growing in importance." Certainly in the case of musculoskeletal medicine, it is the patients' increasing recourse to these therapies that is growing, rather than any intrinsic virtue these may have. These are two distinct matters, their confusion evidence of woolly thinking. On the other hand, the real importance of musculoskeletal medicine lies in the enormous collective incidence of the various problems it addresses, together with the common failure of the medical establishment to meet the challenge that this presents.

It was further noted that "patients themselves are increasingly calling for the use of different forms of treatment." This is true, but such calls are most common where current systems of delivery of conventional medicine are perceived to have failed them or are expected to fail them. This must be taken seriously by the medical profession.

The need to preserve the patient's freedom of choice was stressed, but no mention was made of the necessity that such choice be informed. Proven efficacy and safety must surely be rated higher than unsubstantiated and sometimes frankly invalid diagnostic and therapeutic claims. Very sensibly, reference was made to support not being given to "dubious and intolerant" practices. This is clearly admirable advice, but should it not be extended to dubious and intolerant theories underlying those practices?

The assembly calls for member states to "model their approach on their neighbours' experiments." Without doubt this is wise counsel, provided these experiments have been scrupulously carried out and have been shown to have revealed valid results. The resolution recommends that "appropriate courses should be offered by universities." Yes indeed. But the crucial question has to be which courses are appropriate and how they may be identified. While this aspect was not addressed in this short resolution, it remains essential that courses based on false premises are not included. Nonetheless, this document proceeded to "call on member states to promote official recognition." Prior to any such recommendation being adopted, it is surely mandatory for adequate studies to have been undertaken, reported upon, and discussed – without doctrinaire bias.

Since 1968 the Fédération Internationale de Médecine Manuelle (FIMM) has been the worldwide focus for doctors with an interest in this field. Over the years, its members have produced much original work, some of real scientific merit, in spite of some being less meaningful, while it has moved slowly toward coordination of beliefs, practices, and teaching amongst an increasing number of member associations (45). It is worth noting the widely canvassed, though questionable, view that references to work published more than 10 years ago are insignificant. Surely a logically argued case, challenged year after year without demonstration of invalidity, is more significant than a report as yet inadequately challenged. It is on this basis that scientific knowledge may truly evolve.

As mentioned in the preceding chapter, over the past few years FIMM has undergone significant change. It has radically altered its statutes, expressly to permit the admission to its ranks of organizations previously debarred, by virtue of their memberships not being exclusively medical. I understand that, over this brief period, the membership has increased very considerably. At the same time, of course, FIMM has inevitably rendered itself substantially alternative or complementary. It is no longer exclusively representative of mainstream doctors working in this field. The same considerations apply to the British Institute of Musculoskeletal Medicine (BIMM).

A further matter is of substantial significance: I understand that an European–American Academy of Osteopathy has been set up in Germany, with the express remit to teach this particular alternative to orthodox physicians in Europe. It has to be remembered that osteopathy is fundamentally alternative in origin, theory, and therapeutic intent. This being the case, and in view of the common efficacy and, in the right hands, the remarkable safety of those simple therapeutic procedures outlined in the preceding chapters, it would seem appropriate for the medical establishment now to review the situation as a matter of some urgency.

After all, there is nothing alternative or complementary about vertebral manipulation.

In light of the recommendation of the Parliamentary Assembly (60), it appears that we now have even more reason to reintegrate simple musculoskeletal measures within the compass of the medical establishment, on the sound, scientific bases that have been shown to exist (6), with neither help nor hindrance from any organization that is, by declared intent, not firmly committed to the principles of orthodox medicine. This is a proposition that should appeal to the "new-look"[1] General Medical Council and to deans and staffs of medical schools, as also to interested professional bodies such as the Pain Society. And should not the National Back Pain Association play a part in leaning on the government to implement such improvements?

However, chaos still reigns! It seemed reasonable to hope for an ultimately positive response from the orthodox medical profession following the 2001 conference at the Royal Society of Medicine, "Back Pain – Whose Responsibility?" While this conference was limited to consideration of the lumbar spine, it brought together a number of aspects of the current problem, including some innovative approaches and a sobering view of funding from the Department of Work and Pensions. There was, however, a lamentable paucity of representation of the teaching hospitals, upon whom the profession must rely if it is to provide a more effective service to the patient. Sadly, too little time was set aside for discussion. It is to be hoped that the joint meeting of the Royal Society of Medicine and BIMM that was held in May 2004 has proved to be of greater practical value both to patients and to the medical profession.

However contentious the subject, it seems inescapable that the medical establishment now has the opportunity and the capability to substantially improve the lot of the patient – but only with the abandonment of faith and by publically discarding beliefs which have been shown to be scientifically untenable.

[1]This is a term used by the General Medical Council (GMC) in reference to the recent changes in its statutes and responsibilities.

References

1. Paterson JK, Burn L. (1990) Back Pain – An International Review. London: Kluwer Academic Publishers.
2. Paterson JK. (1997) Report of the Scientific Advisory Committee of the Fédération Internationale de Médecine Manuelle.
3. Wood PHN. (1980) The epidemiology of low back pain. In Jayson, MIV (Ed) Low Back Pain. Tunbridge Wells: Pitman Medical.
4. McNeilly RH, Medical Director, Private Patients Plan, personal communication.
5. Burn L. (1994) A Manual of Medical Manipulation. London: Kluwer Academic Publishers.
6. Burn L, Paterson JK. (1990) Musculoskeletal Medicine: The Spine. London: Kluwer Academic Publishers.
7. British Institute of Musculoskeletal Medicine. Modular course.
8. Paterson JK. (1987) A survey of musculoskeletal problems in general practice. Manuelle Medizin 3:40–48.
9. Paterson JK. (1994) I can tell – an impediment to progress in musculoskeletal medicine. J R Soc Med 87(11):648–649.
10. Maxwell C. (1973) Clinical Research for All. Cambridge: Cambridge Medical Studies.
11. Paterson JK, Burn L. (1990) Basic case analysis. In Paterson JK, Burn L (Eds) Back Pain – an International Review, pp. 64–74. London: Kluwer Academic Publishers.
12. Crombie IK. (1997) Epidemiology of persistent pain. Proceedings of the 8th World Congress on Pain, pp. 53–61. In: Jernsen TS, Turner JA, Weissenfeld-Hallin Z (Eds) Progress in Pain Research and Management, Vol 8. Seattle: IASP Press.
13. Kellgren JH. (1978) In: Copeman WSC (Ed) Textbook of Rheumatic Diseases, 5th ed. London: Pitman Medical.
14. Maigne JY, Maigne R. (1991) Trigger point of the posterior iliac crest; painful iliolumbar ligament insertion or cutaneous dorsal ramus pain? An anatomic study. Arch Phys Med Rehabil 72:734–737.
15. Maigne R. (1992) Douleurs d'Origine Vertébrale et Traitments par Manipulations. Paris: Expansion.
16. Fossgreen J. (1984) Referred pain and tenderness. In: Paterson JK, Burn L (Eds) Back Pain – An International Review. London: Kluwer Academic Publishers, 1990.
17. Wall PD. (1978) The gate control theory of pain mechanisms: a re-examination of statements. Brain 101:1.
18. Wyke B. (1983) Presentation to the 7th Congress of the Fédération Internationale de Médecine Manuelle, Zurich (unpublished).
19. Wall PD. (1979) On the relationship of injury to pain. Pain 6:253–264.
20. Melzack R. (1975) The McGill Pain Questionnaire. Major properties and scoring methods. Pain 1:275–279.

21. Bond MR. (1987) Psychology of pain. In: Anderson S, Bond MR, Mehta M, Swerdlow M (Eds) Chronic Non-cancer Pain. Lancaster: MTP Press.
22. Mixter WH, Barr JS. (1932) Rupture of intervertebral disc with involvement of the spinal cord. N Engl J Med 211:210.
23. Cyriax JH. (1947) Textbook of Orthopaedic Medicine. London: Cassell.
24. Wyke B. (1980) The neurology of low back pain. In: Jayson MIV (Ed) The Lumbar Spine and Low Back Pain, 2nd ed. London: Pitman Medical.
25. Stoddard A. (1966) Manual of Osteopathic Practice. London: Hutchinson & Co.
26. Basmajian JV, DeLuca CJ. (1985) Muscles Alive. Baltimore: Williams & Wilkins.
27. Panjabi M. (1986) Presentation to the 8th International Congress of the Fédération Internationale de Médecine Manuelle, Madrid.
28. Bogduk N. (1997) Musculoskeletal pain; towards precision diagnosis. Proceedings of the 8th World Congress on Pain, pp. 507–525. In: Jensen TS, Turner JA, Weissenfeld-Hallin Z (Eds) Progress in Pain Research and Management, Vol. 8. Congress in Pain Research and Management. Seattle: IASP Press.
29. Palmer DD. (1910) The Chiropractor's Adjustor. Portland, OR.
30. Keith A. (1948) Human Embryology and Morphology. London: Edward Arnold.
31. Clinical Standards Advisory Group. (1994) Report on the Management of Back Pain. London: HMSO.
32. Still AT. (1908) Autobiography. Kirksville, MO.
33. Howitt-Wilson M. (1987) Chiropractic – A Patient's Guide. Wellingborough, England: Thorson's Publishing Group.
34. Wiltze LL. (1971) The effect of the common anomalies of the lumbar spine on disc degeneration in low back pain. Orthop Clin North Am 2:569–582.
35. Torgerson WR, Dotter WE. (1976) Comparative roentgenographics of the asymptomatic and symptomatic spine. J Bone Joint Surg 58:850–853.
36. Collis JL, Ponsetti IV. (1969) Long-term follow-up of patients wit idiopathic scoliosis not treated surgically. J Bone Joint Surg 51:424–455.
37. Hay AC. (1979) The incidence of low back pain in Busselton. In: Twomey LT (Ed) Symposium: Low Back Pain. Perth, Western Australia Institute of Technology Western Australia.
38. Nachemson A. (1980) Lumbar intradiscal pressure. In: Jayson MIV (Ed) The Lumbar Spine and Low Back Pain. Tunbridge Wells, England: Pitman Medical, pp. 341–359.
39. Chaffin DE, Park KS. (1973) A longitudinal study of low back pain associated with occupational weight lifting factors. Am Ind Assoc J 34:531–535.
40. Wilder DG, Woodworth BB, Frymoyer JW, Pope JH. (1982) Vibration and the human spine. Spine 7:243–254.

41. Nicholls PJR. (1960) Short leg syndrome. Br Med J 1:1863.
42. Paterson JK. (1982/83) The lateral index of sacral tilt. Presentations at the congresses of the Fédération Internationale de Médecine Manuelle. Prague and Zurich.
43. Conlon PW, Isdale IC, Rose BS. (1966) Rheumatoid arthritis and the cervical spine. Ann Rheum Dis 25:130.
44. Grisel P. (1930) Enucléation d'atlas et torticollis nasopharyngien. Presse Med 38:50.
45. Paterson JK. (1995) Vertebral Manipulation – A Part of Orthodox Medicine. London: Kluwer Academic Publishers.
46. Koes BW, Assendelft WJJ, van Heijden GJMG, et al. (1991) Spinal manipulation and mobilization for back and neck pain – a blinded review. BMJ 303:298–303.
47. Koes BW, Boulter MM, van Mannever H, et al. (1992) Randomised clinical trial of manipulative therapy and physiotherapy for persistent back and neck complaints – results of 1-year follow-up. BMJ 304:601–605.
48. Meade TW, Dyer S, Brown W, et al. (1990) Low back pain of mechanical origin – randomized comparison of chiropractic and hospital treatment. BMJ 333:431–437.
49. Schekelle PG, Adams AH, Chassin MR, et al. (1992) A review. Spinal manipulation for low back pain. Ann Intern Med 117:590–598.
50. Campbell DG, Parson CM. (1944) Referred head pain and its concomitants. J Nerv Ment Dis 99:544.
51. Magora F, et al. (1944) An electromyographic investigation of the neck muscles in headache. Clin Physiol 14:453.
52. Simons DG, Travell J. (1983) Myofascial pain syndromes. In: Wall PD, Melzack R (Eds) Textbook of Pain. London: Churchill Livingstone.
53. Hitselberger WE, Witten RM. (1968) Abnormal myelograms in asymptomatic patients. J Neurosurg 28:204.
54. Nachemson A. (1976) The lumbar spine: an orthopaedic challenge. Spine 1:59–71.
55. Nachemson A. (1980) In: Jayson MIV (Ed) The Lumbar Spine and Low Back Pain. London: Pitman Medical.
56. British Medical Association. (1986) Report of the Board of Science and Education. Alternative Therapy.
57. Paterson JK, Burn L. (1985) An Introduction to Medical Manipulation. Lancaster: MTP Press.
58. Waddell G, Faber ML, Hutchins PM. (1996) Low Back Pain Evidence Reviewed. London: RCGP.
59. RCGP (Royal College of General Practitioners) Members Reference Book, 2000–2001.
60. Council of Europe Resolution 1206 (1999) of the Parliamentary Assembly.

Further Reading

Basbaum AI, Fields HL. (1984) Endogenous pain control mechanisms. Brainstem pathways and endorphin circuitry. Annu Rev Neurosci 7:309–338.

Basmajian JV. (1980) Muscles and Movements. A Basis for Human Kinesiology. Melbourne, FL: Robert Krieger.

Bergquist-Ullman M, Larsen U. (1977) Acute low back pain in industry. Acta Orthop Scand Suppl 170.

Bond M. (1980) The suffering of severe intractable pain. In Kosterlitz, Terenius (Eds) Pain and Society. Weinheim: Verlag Chemie.

Bonica J. (1953) The Management of Pain. Philadelphia: Lea & Febiger.

Cust G, et al. (1972) The presence of low back pain in nurses. Int Nurse Rev 19:169.

DePoorter AE. (1992) Techniques de Médecine Orthopédique et Manuelle. Les Manipulations Vertébrale. Bruxelles: SRGBMM.

Deyo RA, et al. (1986) How many days of bed rest for low back pain? N Engl J Med 315:1064–1070.

DeLuca C, et al. (1982) Behaviour of human motor units in different muscles during linearly varying contractions. J Physiol 329:113–128.

DuBuisson D, et al. (1979) Amoeboid receptive fields of cells in laminae 1, 2 & 3. Brain Res 177:376–378.

Fields HL, Basbaum AI. (1983) Endogenous pain control mechanisms. In: Wall P, Melzack R (Eds) Textbook of Pain. London: Churchill Livingstone.

Fitzgerald M. (1983) Primary afferents. In: Wall P, Melzack R (Eds) Textbook of Pain. London: Churchill Livingstone.

Gibson HB. (1987) Is hypnosis a placebo? Br J Clin Hypnosis 4:149–155.

Glover J. (1971) Occupational health research and the problem of back pain. Trans Occup Med 21:2.

Grahame R. (1980) Clinical trials in low back pain. Clin Rheum Dis 6:143–156.

Kapandji IA. (1974) Physiology of the Joints, Vol. 3. The Trunk and Vertebral Column. Edinburgh: Churchill Livingstone.

Kirkaldy-Willis WH, Hill RJ. (1979) A more precise diagnosis for back pain. Spine 4:102–109.

Lapsley P. (1990) The economics of back pain. In: Paterson JK, Burn L (Eds) Back Pain, an International Review. London: Kluwer Academic Press.

Lynn B. (1983) The detection of injury and tissue damage. In Wall P, Melzack R (Eds) Textbook of Pain. London: Churchill Livingstone.

Lynn B. (1989) Structure, function and control; afferent nerve endings in the skin. In: Greaves MW, Schuster S (Eds) Pharmacology of the

Skin. Handbook of Pharmacology, Vol 87/1, pp. 175–192. Berlin: Springer-Verlag.

Magora F. (1975) Investigation of the relation between low back pain and occupation. Neurologic and orthopaedic conditions. Scand J Rehabil Med 7:146–151.

Maigne J-Y, Lazaret JP, Guerin Surville H, Maigne R. (1989) The lateral cutaneous branches of the dorsal rami of the thoraco-lumbar junction. An anatomical study on 37 dissections. Surg Radiol Anat 11:289–293.

Maigne J-Y, Doursonian L. (1997) Entrapment neuropathy of the medial superior cluneal nerve. Spine 22:1156–1159.

McMahon SB, Wall PD. (1989) The significance of plastic changes in laminal systems. In: Cervero F, Bennett G, Headley P (Eds) Processing of Information in the Superficial Dorsal Horn of the Spinal Cord. New York: Plenum.

McQuay HA, Moore RA. (1998) An Evidence Based Resource for Pain Relief. Oxford: OUP.

Mehta M. (1987) Simple ways of treating pain. In: Anderson SA, Bond M, Mehta M, Swerdlow M (Eds) Chronic Non-cancer Pain. Lancaster: MYP Press.

Melzack R, Wall P. (1965) Pain mechanisms. A new theory. Science 150:971.

Melzack R, et al. (1977) Trigger points and acupuncture points for pain. Correlation and implication. Pain 3:23.

Nachemson A, Elstrom G. (1970) Intravital dynamic pressure measurements in lumbar discs. A study of common movements, manoeuvres and exercises. Scand J Rehabil Med (Suppl) 1:40.

Nilsonne U, Lundgren A. (1968) Long-term prognosis in idiopathic scoliosis. Acta Orthop Scand 39:456–465.

Noordenboss W. (1983) Prologue. In: Wall P, Melzack R (Eds) Textbook of Pain. London: Churchill Livingstone.

Paterson JK. (1997) Doubting Thomas – his proper role in musculoskeletal medicine. J Musculoskeletal Pain 5(2):117–122.

Piganiol G, et al. (1987) Les Manipulations Vertébrales. Bases Théorique, Clinique et Bioméchanique. Dijon: GEMABFC.

Reading AF. (1989) Testing pain mechanisms in persons in pain. In: Wall P, Melzack R (Eds) Textbook of Pain. London: Churchill Livingstone.

Spangfort E. (1972) The lumbar disc herniation. A computer aided analysis of 2504 operations. Acta Orthop Scand Suppl 142, pp. 1–95.

Waddell G. (1997) Low back pain: a twentieth century care enigma. Proceedings of the 8th World Congress on Pain. In: Jensen TS, Turner JA, Weissenfeld-Hallin Z (Eds) Progress in Pain Research and Management, Vol. 8. Congress in Pain Research and Management. Seattle: IASP Press.

Wyke B. (1980) The neurology of low back pain. In Jayson, MIV (Ed) The Lumbar Spine and Low Back Pain. London: Pitman Medical.

Glossary

A fibres Nerve fibres in peripheral nerves, carrying information other than pain, from their origin in the mechanoceptor end-organs to the dorsal horn of the spinal cord. Also called mechanoceptor fibres.

Annulus fibrosus The tough ring of solid but flexible fibrous tissue surrounding the nucleus pulposus. (*See* intervertebral disc and nucleus pulposus.)

Apophyseal joints *See* posterior vertebral joints.

Atheroma Narrowing of an artery by the deposition of plaques of solid material, largely based on cholesterol. The greater the narrowing, the less the blood flow. There is a possibility of the artery becoming totally blocked, which may be life threatening.

Biomechanics The three-dimensional, mathematical study of movement in humans or other animals.

Bony secondaries Secondary cancerous deposits in bone, derived from primary cancers elsewhere. Apart from causing pain, they may seriously weaken bony structure.

C fibres Relatively small diameter nerve fibres in the same peripheral nerves mentioned under A fibres, carrying pain impulses from their origins in nociceptive end-organs to the basal nuclei of the spinal cord. Pain is felt if the basal nucleus permits onward transmission to the brain. This may be prevented by the simultaneous stimulation of A fibres at the appropriate basal nucleus. Also called nociceptor fibres.

Chiropractic A system of vertebral manipulation based on the belief that many diseases arise from vertebrae or other bones having become displaced. Chiropractic manipulation is specifically intended to replace bones in their proper places.

Cholesterol A normal constituent of blood, derived from saturated fatty acids, such as butter. If raised above the normal level, it increases the risk of deposition of atheromatous plaques. (*See* atheroma.)

Circle of Willis   An anatomical arrangement of arteries that permits transfer of blood from one side of the brain to the other. (*See* vertebral artery occlusion.)

Clinical Standards Advisory Group   A government-sponsored body that in 1994 made a very important report on the management of back pain.

Cranial osteopathy   An offshoot of osteopathy aimed at moving the individual bones of the skull. From childhood, when the bones of the head have stopped growing, these bones are firmly fixed together by bony growth across the sutures, so it is difficult to see how any such movement may be other than imaginary.

Dorsal horn   The area on each side and at every segmental level of the spinal cord where both mechanoceptor and nociceptor fibres terminate, and from which other nerve fibres conduct information to various parts of the brain.

Empirical/empiricism   Experimental/experimentation. A treatment is empirical when there is no clear evidence as to whether it will work or not.

Epidemiology   The study of the natural history of a pathological condition. Who is at risk of getting it? What factors increase or decrease this risk? How is it likely to affect the patient? It is an essential element in planning sensible management.

Facet joints   *See* posterior vertebral joints.

Grisel's syndrome   A condition first described by P. Grisel, in which a child with a sore throat, and for some weeks after recovery from it, may have weakening of the ligaments, which should hold the odontoid process in place. (*See* odontoid process.)

HLA B27   A clearly identified genetic factor associated with rheumatoid arthritis.

Intervertebral disc   The partially solid, partially semifluid structure between two adjacent vertebral bodies, which are of unyielding bone, protected by a thin plate of cartilage. (*See* annulus fibrosus and nucleus pulposus.) For any movement to be possible, the bony parts have to tilt, twist, or slide, or a combination of all three, which means that the nucleus and the annulus are distorted.

Intervertebral joints   The complex of joints, most often three, between adjacent pairs of vertebrae.

Kellgren's "football jersey"   The somewhat crude diagrammatic outline of the surface of the body largely supplied by each segmental nerve. Originally drawn by J.H. Kellgren, he later recognized that this was no more than a rough guide, due to the high degree of overlap in the nerve supply.

McGill Pain Questionnaire   A detailed questionnaire developed for assessing as accurately as possible the degree of pain suffered by the patient.

Mechanoceptors   *See* A fibres.

Mobile segment   Originally described by H. Junghanns, this comprises two neighbouring vertebrae and all the structures keeping them apart, holding them together, and moving one in relation to its neighbour. Of course, no mobile segment ever moves alone, spinal movement invariably being spread over several segmental levels.

Muscle substitution   The phenomenon whereby, in the event of the nerve supply to part of a muscle being damaged (so putting this part out of action), other bundles of muscle fibres, previously at rest, are automatically brought into play. This makes clinical assessment of individual muscle strength extremely difficult.

Neuromuscular system   The system whereby muscle function, which means either its contraction or its relaxation, is governed by a specific part of the nervous system.

Nociceptors   *See* C fibres.

Nucleus pulposus   The inner part of the intervertebral disc. Its importance lies in the fact that, as a semifluid, it cannot be compressed, although it is readily distorted. Its distortion, necessarily coupled with changes in shape and tension in the annulus fibrosus and its supporting ligaments, permits limited movement of the intervertebral joints. When the annulus fibrosus is not adequately contained by its supporting ligaments it will bulge, and the bulge may then press on a nerve root or on the spinal cord. Slight bulging is an essential part of movement, but too great a bulge is known as disc protrusion. If the bulge proceeds to a tear, then rupture of the disc permits irreversible escape of part of the nucleus into the spinal canal.

Odontoid process   The part of the second cervical vertebra that protrudes into the ring of the first cervical vertebra (close to the front), where most of neck rotation takes place. (*See* Grisel's syndrome and rheumatoid arthritis.)

Osteopathy   A system of vertebral manipulation based on the belief that many clinical conditions arise from abnormalities of joint movement, mainly of the spine. Osteopathic manipulation is specifically intended to restore normal joint movement.

Osteoporosis   Structural weakening of bone by demineralization. Commonest in older people, it is related to inadequate calcium intake. Gross osteoporosis may lead to bony fracture as a result of quite minor injury.

Pain modulation   The whole complex of alterations in the nervous system that permits, modifies, or prevents the registration of pain in the brain, or the enhancement of the descending inhibitory pathways of the peripheral nervous system.

Paraesthesia   The pins-and-needles sensation.

Peripheral joints   Joints of the arms and legs.

Pith (verb)   Cause gross damage to the spinal cord in the cervical region.

Posterior vertebral joints   The pairs of joints, sometimes called apophyseal joints, zygoapophyseal joints, or facet joints, behind the vertebral body, between the vertebral arches. (*See* vertebral arch and vertebral body.) Their capsules and supporting ligaments must also be stretched to permit vertebral movement.

Psychosomatic   A symptom derived from both the body and the mind, commonly used in describing pain. Sometimes used in a derogatory manner, but this is ridiculous, as all pain has a beginning in some part of the body, which is modulated in the spinal cord before being recorded in the brain.

"Red flags"   A term used in the CSAG report on back pain to warn the clinician of potential dangers in vertebral manipulation. Applicable to Grisel's syndrome, rheumatoid arthritis, etc.

Referred pain   Pain felt at a distance from its site of origin. Very important in assessing where to apply manipulation or injections.

Referred tenderness   Tenderness felt at a distance from its site of origin. Very important in assessing where to apply manipulation or injections.

Rheumatoid arthritis   A distinct, inflammatory disease, related closely to HLA B27, and certain chemical changes in the blood. A very definite "red flag" for anyone practicing musculoskeletal medicine.

Sacroiliac joints   The pair of joints on either side of the sacrum, attaching the sacrum to the iliac bones. They are the biggest joints in the body, their articular surfaces deeply and irregularly pitted (with prominences to fit the pits) and held together by the strongest ligaments in the body. Contrary to much teaching, the likelihood of damage to these joints is thus remote, and they remain a most unlikely site of origin of pain.

Sacrum   The platform on which the whole spine rests, in order to give attachment to the legs (through the bones of the pelvis.)

Saddle anaesthesia   Loss of sensation in the skin over the sacrum. Not always volunteered by patients, and so they need to be specifically asked about it. Its presence demands immediate surgical referral, as it may progress to serious and permanent disability.

Segmental level   A topographical labeling of the spine, from the first to the seventh cervical vertebrae (C1–C7), through the first to the twelfth thoracic (T1–T12), the first to fifth lumbar (L1–L5), and the first to fifth sacral (S1–S5).

Soma   Body, as distinct from mind.

Somatic Pertaining to the soma.

Spinal canal The channel behind the vertebral bodies, contained posteriorly by the vertebral arches.

Spinal cord The extension of the brain occupying the spinal canal for most of its length, from which the segmental nerve roots arise on either side.

Spinal roots The nerve roots arising segmentally from the spinal cord. It is worth noting that there are seven pairs of cervical roots to six cervical vertebrae; this is due to the first cervical roots really being cranial nerves! Below the end of the spinal cord, the spinal nerve roots continue within the spinal canal, emerging serially at the appropriate lumbar and sacral levels.

Spinous processes The parts of the vertebrae projecting posteriorly and, particularly in the thoracic region, downward, for the attachment of various muscles. It is noteworthy that these are very short in the cervical region, rendering them of no diagnostic use, and that it is uncommon for them to project directly in the midline.

Symphysis pubis The joint between the two pubic bones, joining the pelvis in the front.

Vertebral arch The bones projecting from either side of the vertebral body that curve around to meet each other in the midline, enclosing the spinal canal and forming the base for the spinous processes.

Vertebral artery occlusion Occurs either as a result of gross atheroma or by twisting the neck into a very uncomfortable position and holding this position for some time. This movement may matter, or it may not, depending on the state of the other vertebral artery and the circle of Willis working well.

Vertebral body The solid part of the vertebra, at the front, which gives greatest strength to the spine.

Zygoapophyseal joints *See* posterior vertebral joints.

Index

Page numbers followed by f indicate figures.

A

A fibres, 11
Adrenaline, 81, 84
Anaesthesia
  adverse reactions to, 81
  general, 47, 53, 66
  local, 45, 66, 81–82, 84
  saddle, 33, 69, 73–74, 81
Analgesics, 48
Annulus fibrosus, 13, 75–76
Anterior capsulitis, 61
Apical ligament, 16f
Arteries
  occlusion of, 41–42
  vertebral, 15, 17f, 41–42, 49
Atheroma, 41–42, 49

B

Back pain
  and body posture, 18
  conventional treatment for, 29
  diagnosis of, 12, 46
  epidemiology and mechanisms of, 10
  genetic factors in, 41
  and heavy work, 41, 55–56
  societal costs of, 28, 35
  See also specific areas of spine
Bones. *See specific bones*
Bonesetters, 30–32, 83
Breasts, 64

British Association of Manual Medicine (BAMM), 88
British Institute of Musculoskeletal Medicine (BIMM)
  changes in, 94
  courses sponsored by, 40
  membership of, 2–4
  statutes and history of, 88–91
British Medical Association (BMA), 88–89

C

C fibres, 11
Cancer, bone, 43, 63
Carpal tunnel syndrome, 61
Caudal epidural injections, 45, 81–82, 84
Cervical collars, 58–59
Cervical vertebrae
  cervical ribs, 42
  contraindications to manipulation, 15, 48–54
  headaches arising from, 48
  injections around, 52
  manipulation of, 15, 49–53
  odontoid process of first vertebra, 15, 16f
  and vertebral arteries, 41–42, 49
Chest pain, 63–66
  differential diagnosis of, 63–64
  history-taking in, 64–65
  vertebral manipulation for, 66

Chiropractic/chiropractors
  fees of, 31
  history of, 30, 87
  practices of, 34, 54, 84–85
  terminology of, 29
Clinical Standards Advisory
    Group (CSAG)
  on contraindications, 43
  on need for x-rays, 17
Clinical trials, 46
Coccyx/coccydynia, 74
Coronary artery disease, 63
Costs/cost efficiency
  of misdiagnosis, 36
  to National Health Service
    (NHS), 36–38
  to patients, 85

D

Data recording forms,
    20f–21f, 25f–26f, 33–34
Dermatomal representation,
    10–11
Diagnostic techniques, 19,
    21–24, 43
Doctors/physicians
  costs to/cost efficiency for,
    37
  education/training for, 32,
    35, 38, 90–92
  honesty with patients, 34
  treatment options of, 34–35,
    53, 66
  views of musculoskeletal
    medicine, 32–35, 90
Documentation
  data recording forms,
    20f–21f, 25f–26f, 33–34
  of presenting findings,
    18–21, 25–27, 43, 57
  professional papers
    published, 88–89
Dorsal horn, 12f, 13f

Drugs
  adrenaline, 81, 84
  adverse reactions to, 81
  analgesics, 48
  nonsteroidal anti-
    inflammatory drugs
    (NSAIDs), 60
  steroids, 60–61, 66

E

Ear, nose, and throat (ENT),
    49
ECG (electrocardiography),
    63
Education/training in
  of general practitioners,
    90–92
  for musculoskeletal
    medicine, 6, 38
  for vertebral manipulation,
    45–46, 57
Elbow, 60–62
Electrocardiography (ECG),
    63
Equipment
  of dubious efficacy, 36
  heel lifts, 81
  traction apparatus, 57–58,
    59f, 69–71, 81
ESR (erythrocyte
    sedmentation rate), 60, 65
European–American Academy
    of Osteopathy, 94
Examination, physical
  asymmetrical signs on, 33
  documentation of, 18–21,
    25–27
  orthopaedic and neurologic,
    43

F

Facet joints (posterior
    vertebral)
  anatomy of, 23f

movement of, 14
tenderness in, 43, 74
Fédération Internationale de
    Médecine Manuelle
    (FIMM)
  changes in, 94
  membership of, 2–4
  statutes and history of,
    88–91
Fractures, 43, 60
France, 40
Frontal sinusitis, 48, 50

G
General practitioners
  education/training for,
    90–92
  presenting findings of,
    18–21, 25–27, 43,
    57
Glossary of terms, 101–106
Golfer's elbow, 61
Grisel's syndrome, 42–43,
    52–53

H
Head harness, 57–58, 59f,
    69–71
Headache and migraine,
    48–54
  and asymmetrical physical
    signs, 51–54
  epidemiology and
    symptoms of, 48–50
  unilateral, 48
  vertebral manipulation for,
    48, 51–53
Heel lifts, 81
Herpes zoster, 63
Hippocrates, 2, 32, 86
History-taking, 19, 32–33, 50,
    64–65
Human leukocyte antigen
    (HLA) B27, 41

I
Ilium, 23f, 73, 74
India, 83
Inguinal fossa, 68
Injections
  caudal epidural, 45, 81–82,
    84
  cervical, 52
  for leg pain, 81–82
  peripheral nerve blocks,
    45
  safeguards for, 84
  of steroids, 60–61, 66
  techniques for, 66
  of trigger points, 45, 66,
    81
Interspinous ligament, 14f
Intervertebral discs
  excess pressure on, 75–76
  function of, 12–13
  prolapse of, 64
  protrusion of, 14, 67, 87

J
Joints
  elbow, 60–62
  facet joints (posterior
    vertebral), 14, 23f, 43
  sacroiliac, 42–43, 67, 73
  symphysis pubis, 42–43,
    72

K
Kidneys, 67

L
Labour and delivery, 72,
    74
Lateral index of sacral tilt
    (LIST), 77–81
Leg length, 76–81
  lateral index of sacral tilt
    (LIST) for, 77–81
  x-rays for, 77–79

Leg pain, 75–82
  anterior, 75
  etiology of, 75–76
  injections for, 81–82
  and leg length, 76–81
Ligaments, 14f–16f
  apical, 16f
  longitudinal, 14–16
  pelvic, 42, 73
  strain of, 60–61
  transverse, 16f, 52
  weakening of, 42
Ligamentum flavum, 14f
LIST (lateral index of sacral
    tilt), 77–81
Longitudinal ligament, 14f
Lower trunk pain, 67–71
  history-taking for, 68–69
  prevalence of, 67
  systemic causes of, 67–68
  traction for, 69–71
Lumbago. *See* Lower trunk
    pain
Lumbar spine. *See*
    Thoracolumbar spine

M
Mammals, 12
McGill Pain Questionnaire, 11
Mechanoceptors, 11
Micturition, 69, 73–74, 81
Mobile segments, spinal,
    14–15
Muscles
  guarding, 19, 51
  substitution phenomenom
    in, 15
  tone of paravertebral, 43,
    51, 69, 74
Musculoskeletal medicine
  advantages of, 3, 7, 91–92
  controversy over, 1–4, 9–10,
    89–90
  description of, 1–8

disorders of. *See specific
    disorders*
doctor's view of, 32–35
economics of, 36–39
education/training for, 6,
    32, 35, 38, 40–47, 90–92
efficacy of, 30, 83–85
facilities for, 40
future of, 5–6, 86–92
history of, 4–5, 86–89
manipulative techniques in.
    See Vertebral
    manipulation
patient's view of, 28–31
in primary care, 5, 7, 38–39,
    91–92
professional papers on,
    88–89
prognosis in, 84–85
recognition of, 94–95
scientific bases of, 9–27
Myeloma, 67–68
Myelopathies, 53, 66

N
National Health Service
    (NHS)
  costs to/cost efficiency for,
    36–38
  health care under, 30
  management of, 37
Neck pain, 55–59
  chronic, 55
  and posture, 50
  referred, 56
  traction for, 57–59
Nerves
  compression of, 87
  entrapment of, 68
  fibres of, 10–11, 56
  sciatic, 67, 75
  spinal, 10–11
Neural pathways, 11, 12f–
    13f

Nonsteroidal anti-inflammatory drugs (NSAIDs), 60
Nucleus pulposus, 13, 75

O
Odontoid process, 15, 16f, 42, 52
Osteopathy/osteopaths
  fees of, 31
  history of, 2, 30, 86–87, 94
  manipulative techniques used in, 44
  terminology of, 29
Osteoporosis, 43

P
Pain
  acute and chronic, 11–13, 55
  epidemiology and mechanisms of, 6–7, 40–41
  headache and migraine, 48–54
  mimicking patterns of, 10
  perception of, 41, 56
  psychology of, 11, 53
  radiating, 68
  referred, 10, 33, 56, 73
  terminology of, 7
  with vertebral manipulation, 53, 69, 74
  of vertebral origin (PVO), 40–41, 48, 65
  See also specific body area
Pain of vertebral origin (PVO), 40–41, 48, 65
Palmer, Daniel David, 30, 87
Paravertebral ligaments, 14–16
Patients
  costs to/cost efficiency for, 37, 39, 85
  positioning for manipulation, 44–45
  views of musculoskeletal medicine, 28–31
  wants and needs of, 28–29, 84, 93
Pelvic ligaments, 42, 73
Pelvic pain, 72–74
  etiology of, 72–73
  history-taking for, 73–74
  vertebral manipulation for, 74
Pelvis, 77, 78f–80f
Pericarditis, 63
Peripheral nerve blocks, 45
Physical signs
  asymmetry of, 51–52, 54, 62, 69
  examinations for, 22f–24f
Placebo, 46
Pleurisy, 63
Polymyalgia rheumatica, 60, 65, 67, 73
Posture
  and back pain, 18
  and chest pain, 64
  and neck pain, 50
  at work, 55–56
Primary care
  musculoskeletal medicine in, 5, 7, 38–39, 91–92
  presenting symptoms in, 90
Private Patients Plan, 5
Psychological factors, 11, 53
PVO (pain of vertebral origen), 40–41, 48, 65

R
Radiography. *See* X-rays/radiography
Range of motion (ROM), 50, 56
Resuscitation, 81, 84

Rheumatoid arthritis (RA)
   as a contraindication, 42–43, 66
   as differential diagnosis, 67, 73
   "rheumatoid neck," 52
   treatment for, 60
Ribs, 42, 65
Royal College of General Practitioners (RCGP), 92
Royal Society of Medicine (RSM), 2

S
Sacral thrust, 24f, 74
Sacroiliac joint, 42–43, 67, 73
Sacrum
   anatomy of, 73
   lateral index of sacral tilt (LIST) for, 77–81
   sacral thrust, 24f, 74
Saddle anaesthesia, 33, 69, 73–74, 81
Scar tissue, 82
Scheuermann's disease, 68, 73
Schmorl's nodes, 68
Sciatic nerve, 67, 75
Segmental sagittal pressure, 43, 52, 69, 74
Shoulder and arm pain, 60–62
   differential diagnosis of, 60
   treatment of, 60–61
   vertebral manipulation for, 62
Sit-ups, 76
Skin
   dermatomal representation of pain, 10
   pinching of, 19, 22f–23f, 40–41, 43, 51, 69, 74
Sphincter control, 33
Spinal stenosis, 67
Spine/spinal column
   evolution of, 12

ligaments of, 14f–16f
   mobile segments of, 14–15
   muscles of, 43, 59, 61, 74
   nerves of, 10–11
   See also specific spinal regions
Spinous process pressure (SPP), 19, 22f, 42, 52, 69, 74
Spinous processes, 42
Spreader bars, 69–71
Steroids, 60–61, 66
Still, Andrew Taylor, 30, 87
Studies, clinical, 4, 88–89
Supraspinous ligament, 14f
Surgery, 68, 82
Sympathetic nervous system, 11
Symphysis pubis, 42–43, 72

T
Taxpayers, 36–39
Tenderness, referred, 10, 33, 56, 73
Tennis elbow, 61
Thoracolumbar spine, 68, 72, 74
Tietze's syndrome, 63
Tinnitus, 48–49
Traction, vertebral, 57–58, 59f, 69–71, 81
Transverse ligament, 16f, 52
Trauma
   to head or neck, 48, 55
   to symphysis pubis, 72–73
Trigger points
   injections of, 45, 66, 81
   pressure on, 51
   searching for, 43, 69, 74

U
United Kingdom
   health care in, 30

musculoskeletal medicine
facilities in, 40
population of, 36
practice in, 93

V
Vertebrae
asymmetry of, 51–52, 54, 56
cervical. *See* Cervical
vertebrae
thoracolumbar, 62, 68, 72,
74
Vertebral arteries
cervical, 15, 17f, 41–42, 49
course of, 17f
Vertebral manipulation/
therapeutic techniques
advantages of, 3
cervical, 15, 49–53
choices of, 34–35
contraindications to, 3, 15,
33–34, 41–43, 46, 52–53,
69, 83–84
education/training for, 38,
45–46, 57
efficacy of, 46
for headaches, 48, 51–53
history of, 2, 4

justification for, 17–18
pain with, 53, 69, 74
as placebo, 46
sacral thrust, 24f, 73
thoracolumbar, 62, 66, 68,
72, 74
used in everyday practice,
18, 44
Vertigo/dizziness, 49
Vitreous floaters, 50

W
Whiplash injury, 55
Work, 55–56

X
X-rays/radiography
functional, 17
indications for, 16–17
for leg length test, 77–79

Z
Zygapophyseal joints (Z-
joints)
anatomy of, 23f
movement of, 14
tenderness on pressure, 43,
74